While We Were Sleeping

While We Were Sleeping

Success Stories in Injury and Violence Prevention

David Hemenway

UNIVERSITY OF CALIFORNIA PRESS
Berkeley · Los Angeles · London

University of California Press, one of the most
distinguished university presses in the United States,
enriches lives around the world by advancing
scholarship in the humanities, social sciences, and
natural sciences. Its activities are supported by the UC
Press Foundation and by philanthropic contributions
from individuals and institutions. For more
information, visit www.ucpress.edu.

University of California Press
Berkeley and Los Angeles, California

University of California Press, Ltd.
London, England

Library of Congress Cataloging-in-Publication Data

Hemenway, David, 1945–.

    While we were sleeping : success stories in injury and
violence prevention / David Hemenway.
        p.   cm.
    Includes bibliographical references and index.
    ISBN 978–0–520–25845–7 (cloth : alk. paper)
    ISBN 978–0–520–25846–4 (pbk. : alk. paper)
    1. Accidents—Prevention—History—United States.
2. Accidents—Prevention—Government policy—
United States   I. Title.
    [DNLM: 1. Accident Prevention—history—
United States.   2. Consumer Product Safety—United
States.   3. Government Regulation—United States.
4. Protective Devices—United States.   5. Violence—
prevention & control—United States.   6. Wounds and
Injuries—prevention & control—United States. WA 11
AA1 H488w 2009]
HV675.H46   2009
362.197′107—dc22   2008028117

Manufactured in the United States of America

18   17   16   15   14   13   12   11   10   09
10   9   8   7   6   5   4   3   2   1

This book is printed on Natures Book, which contains
30% post-consumer waste and meets the minimum
requirements of ANSI/NISO Z39.48–1992 (R 1997)
(*Permanence of Paper*).

For Michelle and the Hemenways

Contents

Tables

Preface

As a child, my favorite fairy tale was "The Elves and the Shoemaker." As told by the Brothers Grimm, it went something like this: There once was a poor shoemaker who worked very hard, but he still could not earn enough to live on, until at last all he had was just enough leather to make one pair of shoes. He cut the leather out and went to bed. In the morning, to his great wonder, he awoke to find the shoes already made. The workmanship was wonderful, and he was able to sell the shoes at a high price. With the money, he bought leather enough for two pairs of shoes. He cut the leather out and went to bed. In the morning he found two pairs of perfectly made shoes. These were also sold at a high price, and he had enough money to buy leather for four pair of shoes. And so it went. Pretty soon the shoemaker became rich. One evening the shoemaker hid, and around midnight in came two little elves. They sat upon the shoemaker's bench, took the work that was cut out, and began to ply their little fingers, stitching and rapping and tapping at such a rate until the job was done.

I still love that fairy tale, the idea of the elves coming to make the shoemaker's life better. Public health practitioners, like the elves, are people who try to make my life, and yours, better—usually without our knowing who they are. This book is written to acknowledge those public health workers who have made important contributions to safety and health by helping to reduce injuries and violence "while we were sleeping."

Over the past century there have been many successes in injury prevention; injury rates have fallen substantially in the United States and in other developed countries. Yet injuries remain a major public health problem. In 2005 more than 173,000 Americans died from injuries, and there were almost 30 million nonfatal emergency department visits for injury. Indeed, the majority of Americans who die between the ages of 1 and 40 die from injury, not disease. Injury deaths in the United States account for more lost years of productive life before the age of 65 than heart disease, cancer, and stroke combined.

Injury events occur when energy transfer results in tissue damage. The five forms of energy are kinetic (e.g., car crash), chemical (e.g., poisoning), thermal (e.g., burns), electrical (e.g., lightning strike), and radiation (e.g., x-rays). There are many types of injury, resulting, for example, from falls, drowning, fire, repetitive motion, whiplash, sports, natural disasters, rape, child abuse, self-harm, and assault, and there are many ways to reduce injury. One reason to assemble a large collection of success stories is to illustrate the wide variety of approaches that can benefit society.

This book contains over sixty success stories. The criterion for inclusion was the clear demonstration of either a quantifiable reduction in injuries or an important intermediate outcome (e.g., seat belt use, smoke detector availability) that should reduce injuries. While I believe the scientific evidence for the successes is quite convincing, almost every issue has some controversy; for example, although there are dozens of peer-reviewed journal articles (e.g., Houston & Richardson 2008; Chenier & Evans 1987) showing the injury reduction benefits of motorcycle helmet laws, a quick search of the Internet finds many biker sites denying the evidence.

The successes are not always due to actions of self-proclaimed injury-control professionals or even of public health officials. They include actions by individuals, employers, nonprofits, and government agencies. Tort lawsuits provide the impetus for some of the beneficial initiatives.

Many safety features (e.g., faucets that mix hot and cold water to reduce scalds) undoubtedly are beneficial, but are not included as a success story unless there is statistical evidence of benefit. Many "best practices" are also not included because they have not been sufficiently tested on a wider population (e.g., breakaway bases that reduce sliding injuries in softball).

The stories are not necessarily the most important successes; the goal was to provide a wide range of inspiring examples. The success stories in this book explain only a small part of the reduction in injuries in the past century. More could almost always be done; even these success stories are rarely complete successes.

The success stories are longitudinal, examining what happened to injury rates over time. The book does not include successes suggested by cross-sectional comparisons (e.g., compared with the United States, all the other developed countries have succeeded in having much lower levels of firearm violence). Also not included are those injury success stories that are difficult to document but are perhaps the most important: preventing a danger before any injury occurs. For example, in the 1980s some firearm manufacturers began making guns with more plastic and less metal. Such guns are more likely to be mistaken for toys, and, when disassembled, these guns are more difficult to detect with metal detectors in courtrooms, prisons, airports, and elsewhere. A 1988 federal law required that all guns sold in the United States contain a minimum amount of metal. There is now little profit to be made by further development of a plastic firearm, and it is unlikely that an all-plastic firearm will be produced commercially or made widely available. The law prevented what might (or might not) have developed into a serious public health problem.

The book divides the success stories into seven categories: car, home, work, play, nature, violence, and medical treatment. In addition there is a chapter on models for success, examining an industry, a town, a city, and two countries. There is also a chapter on successes for the future (i.e., current failures). Indeed, it would have been much easier to write a book on failures in injury and violence prevention than on successes. There is still much work to be done.

Each of the seven categories contains examples of heroes of injury prevention, people who have made a difference in making the world safer. These heroes demonstrate that the actions of individuals can dramatically improve the safety of large numbers of people. While I believe strongly in the importance of research in promoting safety, I decided to write mostly about activists rather than researchers. I selected the activists not only because what they did is important, but because how they did it appealed to me and suggested lessons for future advocates. A different author might have made a somewhat different selection of heroes.

The few paragraphs in this book about each hero (and each success story) provide only a brief summary, emphasizing some of the highlights of his or her accomplishments. It is obviously not the full and complete story. One could well write a book about each success and each hero.

The success stories and heroes do not include examples of preventing injury by preventing or stopping wars (Mathews 2002). Thus my father's hero, five-star general George Marshall, whose Marshall Plan began the post–World War II reconstruction plan of Europe, which earned him the Nobel Peace Prize in 1953, is not included.

The success heroes in this book are individuals rather than institutions. While not the focus of this book, it should be emphasized that many government agencies, corporations, and nonprofit institutions have played, and continue to play, crucial roles in reducing injury in the United States and the world. A small sample from the very long list of U.S. institutions that deserve accolades include, at the federal level, the Centers for Disease Control and Prevention, the Consumer Product Safety Commission, the National Institute for Occupational Safety and Health, and the National Traffic Highway Safety Administration; at the state and local level, public health agencies, fire departments, and law enforcement; nonprofits such as the American Society for Testing and Materials, the Society of Automotive Engineers, the National Safety Council, Underwriters' Laboratories, the National Fire Protection Association, the Insurance Institute for Highway Safety, the ECRI Institute, and the Institute for Healthcare Improvement. Many for-profit companies have also been in the vanguard of reducing injury by making safer products and safer workplaces.

My personal interest in injury prevention began in the 1960s, when I worked for Ralph Nader and for Consumers' Union. I wrote my economics dissertation on voluntary standards (which often form the basis for mandatory safety standards).

In the 1970s I taught economics to undergraduates at Harvard, Boston University, and Wellesley College before teaching a course at Harvard School of Public Health (HSPH). I knew almost nothing about public health, but I fell in love with the HSPH students; their median age was 31 (my age), about one-third were doctors, and one-third were international students. They were intelligent and motivated. They had already received a good education and been blessed in many other ways, and they wanted to give something back to society. Economics was something they needed to know; I was teaching them something important for their careers. I tried to figure out a way to stay in public health.

In the early 1980s I wrote a book on inspection (mostly inspections about safety) and created a course at HSPH dealing directly with safety, Introduction to Injury Prevention. I was warned that injury prevention was not really public health; fortunately for me, in 1986 America's leading public health agency, the Centers for Disease Control (CDC), proclaimed that injury was indeed an important (and neglected) public health problem. There were funds to support my research.

Over the past two decades I have been working at the Harvard Injury Control Research Center, whose core funding is provided by a grant from the CDC. The CDC also supported part of this project, and Harvard School of Public Health gave me an eight-month sabbatical that enabled me to finish the book.

This book is my personal ode to public health. Public health is pragmatic and optimistic, and one goal of the book is to impart some of that optimism. Public health, and public health practitioners, can and have made a difference.

While I was writing this book I tried hard to think about my intended audience. I want my book to be useful to all interested readers, but I decided that one group of particular importance was the parents of my students. When my students were deciding to return to school in public health their parents would often ask, "Now, what exactly is public health?," and the students would rarely have an easy answer. I want them to be able to say, "Here, read this book."

Many people helped me on this project. I would like especially to thank Deb Azrael, Susan Baker, Cathy Barber, Renee Johnson, Matthew Miller, Michelle Schaffer, Alix Smullin, and Sara Solnick. Erin Burke, Steven Lippmann, and especially Coppelia Liebenthal helped me gather materials. My students in Principles of Injury Prevention provided some of the success stories and heroes.

Introduction

In 1900 the average life expectancy of Americans was 47 years. Today it is 78 years. Most of this improvement in health has been due to public health measures rather than medical advances (Evans, Barer, & Marmor 1994). Unfortunately, most Americans do not have a good understanding of public health.

How does the public health approach differ from the medical approach? Public health does not deal directly with individuals, but with populations. Unlike the case-by-case approach of much of medicine, the concern of public health is to improve the health of societies. As the motto of the Johns Hopkins School of Public Health proclaims, "Protecting Health, Saving Lives—*Millions at a Time.*"

Unlike medicine, the focus of public health is not on cure, but on prevention. And unlike criminal justice, the goal is neither to find fault, to assign blame, nor to punish offenders (though punishment to prevent health problems from arising is one aspect of the public health approach). The real goal of public health is to eliminate the danger before something bad happens.

The scientific underpinning of public health is epidemiology, which identifies risk factors, trends, and causes of health problems. But sound science is only the beginning of the public health approach. Public health officials are also advocates for policies that improve society's well-being. Rallying social and political support for feasible solutions is the way public health has achieved many beneficial results.

One of the most important public health advances of the nineteenth century was the "great sanitary awakening," which found that filth was both a cause of disease and a vehicle of transmission (Winslow 1923). Sanitation forever altered the way society thought about health; instead of seeing illness as an indicator of poor moral or spiritual conditions, we began to understand that some illnesses were a result of poor environmental conditions. Public health emphasized the need to change the environment as well as individual behavior.

Attempts in the nineteenth century to combat tuberculosis were successful largely because they addressed poor sanitation and overcrowding in urban neighborhoods, rather than because of individual medical treatments (Haines 1997). Recognition that environmental and social conditions were crucial in leading to disease outbreaks meant that health could no longer be considered solely the responsibility of the individual.

For most of human history injuries were regarded as random and unavoidable events or retribution for human evil or carelessness. They were accidents or acts of God. The main strategies for prevention were prayer or human improvement (e.g., moral education and punishment). In the nineteenth century, industrialization and the public health movement combined to emphasize the importance of environmental factors leading to injury.

Throughout the twentieth century, corporations and government increasingly recognized the importance of their policies in determining rates of injury. For example, the industrial Safety First movement of the 1920s helped focus attention on the role of the employer in ensuring worker safety. A burst of federal activity in the late 1960s and early 1970s establishing federal agencies to promote traffic safety, consumer product safety, and occupational safety was a twentieth-century milestone, as was the emergence in the mid-1980s of injury science as a distinct field of research within the domain of public health (Institute of Medicine 1999).

Over the past century, many advances have been made in reducing injury. For example, the unintentional injury death rate in the United States fell from 116 per 100,000 people in 1930 to 40 per 100,000 in 2005. Today much scientific research is conducted to better understand and further reduce injuries and violence. The appendix discusses scientific injury prevention studies and provides a small sample of the types of studies published in peer-reviewed journals in 2005. The appendix illustrates the wide variety of injuries and the types of knowledge that will help to suggest and evaluate interventions that may increase our safety.

Public health often meets with organized opposition. The "sanitary idea"—building a drainage network to remove sewage and waste—was quite controversial in the nineteenth century. In the twentieth century, campaigns to reduce the public health burden caused by such factors as tobacco, alcohol, and obesity provoked powerful social and economic interests. Past and current efforts to reduce the heavy injury toll also often meet with fierce opposition (e.g., motor cycle helmet laws, gun control laws).

A public relations problem for public health is that most people do not recognize, or do not readily recall, when they personally have benefited from a public health intervention. The consumer who does not get poisoned because unsafe products are kept off the market does not even know that her life has been saved as a result of the efforts of the public health community. Similarly, few people know of the public health heroes who make our lives so much safer. One purpose of this book is to raise awareness of some of the benefits provided by public health.

Public health has many success stories, including the elimination of smallpox (which killed my grandfather) and the reduction of other infectious diseases. U.S. public health success stories during my lifetime include the reduction in cigarette smoking, the removal of much dog poop in cities, and the improvement in the quality of air and water in most urban areas. Public health also has many heroes, men and women who have made a difference. They include Albert Schweitzer, Mother Teresa, and John Snow. Everyone knows about the first two, and Dr. John Snow is well known to almost everyone in public health. During the London cholera epidemic of 1854, Dr. Snow identified the cause of the outbreak as the public water pump on Broad Street; the removal of the pump handle helped stop the spread of the disease. Snow's use of statistics to illustrate the connection between water quality and cholera cases is often regarded as the founding event in the science of epidemiology ("John Snow" 2005).

Unfortunately most public health heroes are not well known. In this book I tell the stories of individuals, many of whom you may not recognize, who have made a difference in preventing injuries. They are not presented as the most important injury prevention figures, but their stories help illustrate the activities undertaken to promote public health and safety. Many people are alive today, or uninjured today, because of the dedication of such people. Their stories show that single individuals and groups of individuals can make a tremendous difference in all our lives.

The poem that follows was written more than a century ago. It illustrates a key concept of public health: that injury prevention is better than cure. Unfortunately that simple idea is still too often ignored in the real world when scarce resources are being allocated.

The Ambulance in the Valley

Joseph Malins, 1895

'Twas a dangerous cliff, as they freely confessed,
Though to walk near its crest was so pleasant;
But over its terrible edge there had slipped
A duke, and full many a peasant.
The people said something would have to be done,
But their projects did not at all tally.
Some said "Put a fence 'round the edge of the cliff,"
Some, "An ambulance down in the valley."

The lament of the crowd was profound and was loud,
As their tears overflowed with their pity;
But the cry for the ambulance carried the day
As it spread through the neighboring city.
A collection was made, to accumulate aid,
And the dwellers in highway and alley
Gave dollars and cents—not to furnish a fence—
But an ambulance down in the valley.

"For the cliff is all right if you're careful," they said;
"And, if folks ever slip and are dropping,
It isn't the slipping that hurts them so much
As the shock down below—when they're stopping."
So for years (we have heard), as these mishaps occurred
Quick forth would the rescuers sally,

To pick up the victims who fell from the cliff,
With the ambulance down in the valley.

Said one, in a plea, "It's a marvel to me
That you'd give so much greater attention
To repairing results than to curing the cause;
You had much better aim at prevention.
For the mischief, of course, should be stopped at its source;
Come, neighbors and friends, let us rally.
It is far better sense to rely on a fence
Than an ambulance down in the valley."

"He is wrong in his head," the majority said,
"He would end all our earnest endeavor.
He's a man who would shirk this responsible work,
But we will support it forever.
Aren't we picking up all, jut as fast as they fall,
And giving them care liberally?
A superfluous fence is of no consequence
If the ambulance works in the valley."

But a sensible few, who are practical too,
Will not bear with such nonsense much longer;
They believe that prevention is better than cure,
And their party will soon be much stronger.
Encourage them then, with your purse, voice and pen,
And while other philanthropists dally,
They will scorn all pretense and put up a stout fence
On the cliff that hangs over the valley.

Better guide well the young, than reclaim them when old,
For the voice of true wisdom is calling,
"To rescue the fallen is good, but 'tis best
To prevent other people from falling."
Better close up the source of temptation and crime
Than deliver from dungeon or galley
Better put a strong fence 'round the top of the cliff
Than an ambulance down in the valley.

CHAPTER 1

Car

INTRODUCTION

Motor vehicle fatalities are the leading cause of injury death in every developed nation. In 2005 in the United States 120 people died per day in traffic crashes, and traffic crashes were the leading cause of death for every age from 2 through 34. Motor vehicle crashes also cause nonfatal serious injury, such as traumatic brain injury and spinal cord injury. On an average day in 2005, over 9,000 Americans were injured seriously enough in traffic crashes to seek medical attention in hospital emergency departments.

Fortunately many policies can help reduce traffic injuries. Using a matrix (Table 1) developed by Bill Haddon, we can first divide policies into three categories: those focused on (1) the human (e.g., the driver), (2) the vehicle, and (3) the road. We can also divide policies into three categories: those focused on (a) the pre-event (preventing the collision), (b) the event (reducing the immediate harm caused by the collision), and (c) the postevent (ameliorating the injury and preventing further injury).

The first seven success stories in this section focus on the human, and the first three deal with policies that attempt to reduce alcohol-related injuries. Alcohol consumption is a risk factor for serious automotive injury; indeed, it is a risk factor for virtually every type of injury. Policies that raise the minimum legal drinking age, increase the likelihood of being caught drunk driving, and raise the penalties for being caught are designed primarily to reduce the chances of a crash by changing driver

TABLE I
Haddon matrix

	Human	Vehicle (agent of injury)	Environment
Pre-event	1	4	7
Event	2	5	8
Postevent	3	6	9

behavior (Cell 1 in Table 1). The focus is on the pre-event. In addition, alcohol in the body tends to increase the seriousness of injury once a collision has occurred. It is a myth that a drunk person is less likely to be injured during a crash or fall because relaxed. The evidence shows conclusively that in the same collision a drunk individual is far more likely to be injured severely than others who have not been drinking (Evans 2004). The fourth success story (graduated driving licenses) deals with policies that focus on the pre-event and are designed to reduce injuries to the young, inexperienced driver.

In the next three success stories, the focus is on changing human behavior to reduce the seriousness of injury once the collision has occurred (Cell 2). The goal is to reduce the injuries caused by the "second collision," when the human body decelerates into the interior of the vehicle or some other object. Seat belts, helmets, and child safety seats do little to reduce the likelihood of collisions but protect the human during the event (crash) phase of the incident. However, the occupant must take appropriate action for the devices to have a beneficial effect: the motorist has to "buckle up," to wear the motorcycle helmet, or to strap a child into the child safety seat.

Some of the most important changes in motor vehicle safety in the past half-century have been safety improvements to the vehicle itself. These improvements include better headlights and brakes, energy-absorbing steering columns and laminated front windshields, head rests (reducing whiplash injuries), seat belts with shoulder straps, and air bags. Some of these changes reduce the likelihood of collision (e.g., headlights, brakes; Cell 4); some primarily reduce the likelihood of immediate injury once the collision occurs (e.g., air bags, steering column and windshield improvements; Cell 5); and some reduce the likelihood of subsequent injury (e.g., improvements in gas tanks that lessen the likelihood of fire after the collision; Cell 6). Many of these changes are "passive" safety measures; that is, they do not require the motorist to do anything to be protected.

In the United States in the late 1960s and early 1970s the forerunner of the National Highway Safety Administration mandated many safety standards for new motor vehicles. It is estimated that by 1980 these standards had reduced occupant deaths by some 40 percent (Crandall et al. 1986). Virtually all developed countries now have similar safety standards for automobiles.

Three success stories in this section deal with changes in the motor vehicle. The third brake light reduces the likelihood of collision (Cell 4), and energy-absorbing steering columns and air bags reduce the likelihood that the second collision will cause serious injury (Cell 5). An additional success story deals with the gasoline that is used to power the vehicle; getting the lead out of gasoline reduces the likelihood of lead poisoning to people in the community.

Roads are much better than they were a half-century ago, reducing the likelihood of collision (e.g., better lighting; Cell 7) and the seriousness of a collision (e.g., deformable lampposts; Cell 8). Sometimes road improvements do both; for example, improved guardrails keep an out-of-control motorist from crashing into other cars or unmovable objects and make it less likely that the motorist will suffer serious injury from colliding with the guardrail itself (Cell 8).

Speed bumps cause motorists to slow down and thus protect pedestrians and other vehicles (Cell 7). Indeed, there a score of other "traffic calming" road measures, including chicanes (road narrowings that alternate from one side of the street to the other, forming S-shaped curves) and neckdowns (sidewalk extensions at intersections that reduce roadway width from curb to curb), which help keep pedestrians safe (Elvik 2001). At the extreme, one way to protect pedestrians is to ban motor vehicles entirely from an area, as by the creation of pedestrian streets.

The final three success stories in this chapter deal with measures that change the roadway. Roundabouts and guardrails reduce both the likelihood and the seriousness of injury (Cells 7 and 8). Crash cushions largely reduce the severity of injury once the collision has occurred (Cell 8). These are three of the many types of road improvements that have made driving so much safer (but still not safe enough).

The Centers for Disease Control and Prevention (CDC) calls the improvements in traffic safety in the United States a "twentieth century public health achievement" (CDC 1999). The creation of an excellent data system by the National Highway Traffic Safety Administration enabled scientists to determine the main factors affecting road safety and which public policies were and were not effective (Waller 2002). Yet many areas for improvement still exist, particularly concerning teens and elderly drivers.

CAR SUCCESS STORIES

1.1. Minimum Legal Drinking Age

Injuries are the leading cause of death for youths ages 18–20, and alcohol is a risk factor for sustaining a fatal injury. Historically, the minimum legal drinking age in the United States has ranged from 18 to 21. In the 1970s and 1980s numerous state legislatures enacted changes to the drinking age. In 1970, thirty-three states had a drinking age of 21; between 1970 and 1975, twenty-five state legislatures lowered their drinking age to 18. Starting in 1977 many states began raising the legal drinking age, until by 1988 the minimum legal drinking was 21 in all states.

This natural experiment is the most well-studied alcohol control policy in U.S. history. At least forty-six high-quality studies find an inverse relationship between the drinking age and traffic crashes among youths 18 to 20 years old: when the drinking age goes down, traffic injuries and fatalities among youth go up, and vice versa. The relationship holds even when there has not been strong enforcement of the law and youth still have some access to alcohol. The National Highway Traffic Safety Administration estimates that traffic fatalities have fallen by over 800 deaths per year due to the higher drinking age. Raising the legal drinking age to 21 probably also reduced other injuries; one study found an 8 percent reduction in youth suicides when the drinking age rose from 18 to 21.

> LESSON: Laws can have a beneficial effect, even when there is little enforcement and some people flout the law.

1.2. Random Breath Testing

Alcohol consumption substantially increases the risk of a motor vehicle crash. In 1982 in New South Wales, Australia, police introduced highly visible checkpoints on main thoroughfares, and passing drivers were chosen arbitrarily and directed to stop for an alcohol breath test. Implementation of the program was intensive. Two hundred new highway patrolmen were recruited to help administer the tests. By the end of the fifth year of operation, over 50 percent of the motorists in Sydney had been tested at least once, and 80 percent reported seeing the program in operation. The campaign received extensive publicity and included a catchy jingle: "How will you go when you sit for the test, will you be under .05 or under arrest?"

The intervention led to a sustained decrease in motor vehicle fatalities of some 15 to 20 percent due to a reduction in alcohol-related crashes. "This is one of the clearest and largest changes in traffic safety associated with a specific intervention" (Evans 2004, 254). The effects were credited more to deterrence than to catching motorists driving drunk. Four elements of the campaign helped ensure its success: publicity, visibility, enforcement, and sustainability. Random breath testing has been widely adopted in other Australian states, with comparable results.

LESSON: Enforcement of the law is one way (but not the only way)
          of reducing dangerous behavior.

1.3. Increased Penalties for Drunk Driving

Alcohol-impaired driving is a leading cause of traffic fatalities in developed and developing countries. In 2002 Japan enacted a law designed to reduce alcohol-impaired driving. The law reduced the allowable blood alcohol concentration from .05 percent to .03 percent. More important, it substantially increased the penalties. Fines for drunk driving were raised from $425 to $4,250, a tenfold increase. In addition, the law made bartenders and passengers culpable along with the arrested drivers.

The new law was widely publicized. The official advertisement for the campaign was memorable. In it, a drunken man intends to go home in his car, and the bartender requests that he pay $4,250 for the last drink, equal to the drunk-driving penalty and more than the average monthly salary in Japan.

The law appears to have been quite successful. Comparing the period before and after the law, alcohol-impaired traffic fatalities fell 38 percent (all traffic fatalities fell 14 percent), and alcohol-impaired serious traffic injury fell 37 percent (all severe traffic injury fell 4 percent). These large reductions occurred even though the definition of alcohol-impaired driving was expanded in the postlaw period, including drivers with .03 percent and .04 percent blood alcohol concentrations.

LESSON: Substantially increased penalties for dangerous behavior
          can sometimes help prevent injury.

1.4. Graduated Driver's Licenses

Sixteen-year-olds have almost ten times the crash risk of drivers ages 30–59 and close to three times the risk of older teenagers. A contributor to the elevated risk is lack of driving experience, but the best way to get experience is by driving. What is needed is a way to gain experience while minimizing risk. This is the goal of graduated licensing.

Graduated licensing is designed to phase in on-road driving, permitting novices to gain experience under safer conditions. The first few months of driving have the highest crash rates. Early research also identified the overrepresentation of young drivers in crashes at night and when another young person was the right front passenger.

A graduated license system typically entails a six-month supervised learner's permit (e.g., with a minimum of fifty hours certified driving), followed by an intermediate phase that permits unsupervised driving only in less risky situations (e.g., during the day and with no other adolescents in the car, unless accompanied by an adult). Full licensure follows if all the conditions of the first two stages have been met.

In 1984 New Zealand became the first country to adopt a graduated licensing system. Michigan became the first U.S. state, in 1997. By 2006 some elements of graduated licensing had been adopted in all fifty states. The reductions in crash and injury rates among 16- and 17-year-olds have been impressive. For example, crash risk among 16-year-old Michigan drivers fell 29 percent between 1996 and 2001. A review article of the more than two dozen evaluations of graduated licensing systems for the United States and Canada concluded, "The results [of all the studies] are surprisingly consistent. Overall, graduated driver licensing programs have reduced the youngest drivers' crash risk by roughly 20 to 40%" (Shope 2007, 165).

> LESSON: Research can help identify risk factors for injury and help inform sensible policy.

1.5. Seat Belt Use

The efficacy of seat belts in reducing mortality and morbidity in traffic crashes has been well established. A problem has been getting motorists to buckle up. In 1980, for example, only 11 percent of the U.S. motoring population wore seat belts. By 1999 that percentage had increased to 71, a clear injury prevention success story. The National Highway Traffic Safety Administration estimates that seat belts probably saved more than 11,000 lives in 1999 alone.

The big jump in U.S. seat belt use came between 1984 and 1992, when usage rates went from 14 to 62 percent. In 1984 the U.S. secretary of transportation ruled that passive restraints (e.g., air bags) would not be required in motor vehicles if more than two-thirds of the nation's population resided in states with mandatory seat belt laws meeting five specific criteria. The auto industry, which had long fought passive restraint requirements for their vehicles, immediately began a massive lobbying campaign to enact state seat belt laws, forming a new organization, Traffic Safety Now, to spearhead the effort. No state had a seat belt law in 1983; by the time Traffic Safety Now closed its doors in 1992, forty-two states had enacted seat belt laws. In an ironic twist for the auto companies, but of great benefit for safety, it was ruled that many of the state laws did not satisfy the criteria in the regulation, and the United States ended up with both state seat belt laws and automobile air bags.

LESSON: Given the right incentive, industry can often push
             successfully for laws promoting consumer safety.

1.6. Helmet Laws

Taiwan has one of the highest motorcycle use rates in the world; over two-thirds of their motor vehicles are motorcycles. In mid-1997 Taiwan followed most other Asian countries by enacting a mandatory helmet use law for cyclists. Mandatory helmet laws are easily enforced because noncompliance is readily observed. Helmet use rose immediately, from about 20 percent to over 95 percent; the number of licensed cyclists remained the same. In the first six months following the law, fatalities due to motorcycle head injuries fell 22 percent (all motorcycle-related deaths fell 14 percent) and nonfatal head injuries fell 44 percent. Although the vast majority of cyclists wore helmets, over half of all motorcycle-related head injuries were to individuals who were not wearing a helmet.

One of the beneficial side effects of motorcycle helmet laws is that they reduce motorcycle theft. For example, following the mandatory helmet law in West Germany in 1980, while thefts of cars and bicycles remained largely unchanged, motorcycle thefts fell from 153,000 in 1980 to 54,000 in 1986. Why the reduction? It turned out that many thefts were opportunistic rather than carefully planned. Any would-be thief who had not brought along a helmet would be quickly noticed by the police and pulled over for violating the helmet law. Similarly, in London, motorcycle thefts fell 24 percent after Great Britain enacted a helmet law in 1973, and the Netherlands saw a 36 percent drop in thefts in 1975 when its law was enacted.

> LESSON: Regulations of observable conduct typically have a larger
> effect than regulations of unobservable conduct.

1.7. Child Safety Seats

In the 1960s it was common for parents to hold their infant in their lap while traveling in a motor vehicle. During a crash, the physical forces would make it impossible to keep hold of the child, who would fly through the air, crashing into the inside of the car or through the windshield. Often the child would serve as an "air bag" for the parent who was supposedly protecting her.

In the 1970s the major policy initiatives in child passenger safety were educational. When it became clear that education alone was not sufficiently changing parental behavior, a small group of pediatricians in Tennessee lobbied that parents be required by law to restrain small children in their cars. The lobbying was effective: some legislators were approached by the very pediatrician who cared for his or her children. In 1978 Tennessee became the first state to mandate child safety seat use. Between 1978 and 1983 in Tennessee, occupant deaths to children under age 4 declined by more than 50 percent. Children not in a restraint device were eleven times more likely to die in a crash than those who were restrained.

By 1985 every state had passed child seat restraint legislation. Safety seat use in cities rose from 23 percent in 1982 to 82 percent in 1987.

> LESSON: A few determined people can save many lives.

1.8. Third Brake Light

Rear-impact collisions account for more than 20 percent of all motor vehicle crashes. In 2005, for example, it was estimated that there were more than 1.2 million rear-impact crashes involving passenger cars, with 400,000 injured occupants. Countermeasures intended to reduce the problem have included head restraints, crash-resistant gasoline tanks, stronger bumpers—and improved brake lights. Between 1977 and 1980 fleets of taxicabs and telephone company passenger cars were randomly provided with center, high-mounted brake lights. The cars so fitted were rear-ended 44 to 54 percent fewer times while braking than those cars without this third brake light.

Based on these randomized studies the National Highway Traffic Safety Administration required that all passenger cars manufactured after August 1985 be equipped with a center high-mounted stop lamp. Studies find that these lights have reduced rear-end collisions, but only by 4 to 5 percent. Part of the reason for the lower levels of effectiveness is that drivers may have become acclimated to the new lights, and the novelty effect has worn off. Still, even a 4 percent reduction in rear-end collisions may represent some 25,000 injuries prevented each year.

> LESSON: Safety devices work, but sometimes have less of a real-
> world impact than predicted.

1.9. Energy-Absorbing Steering Columns

The steering assembly is the most common source of serious injury for drivers in frontal crashes. In most passenger cars before the 1967 model year the steering column was a rigid pole ending in a narrow hub. It was like a spear pointed at the chest of the driver. In frontal crashes, the driver would hit the rigid column with the force concentrated on the narrow hub. Even worse, the steering column would often be propelled rearward, toward the driver, at a high rate of speed. Not surprisingly, the driver's lungs and other internal organs would be punctured, and the driver would often die.

In the 1960s the General Services Administration began requiring improved steering assemblies in government-purchased vehicles. In 1967 the new National Highway Traffic Safety Administration extended this requirement to all new passenger cars sold in the United States. A comprehensive analysis of the safety benefits estimated that these safer steering assemblies reduced the risk of driver fatality in a frontal crash by 12 percent and the risk of serious injury to the driver by over 17 percent. For 1978 alone, that meant 1,300 fewer driver deaths and 24,200 fewer serious injuries. The average cost to the consumer for this safety feature was only $10.50 per car. Most motorists were unaware of this important safety improvement.

> LESSON: Many important public health policies can benefit
> consumers without their awareness.

1.10. Government Purchase of Air Bags

Government-mandated motor vehicle air bags are currently saving the lives of thousands of motorists each year. The struggle to ensure that motor vehicles were equipped with such passive restraint systems was a long and tortuous one. One step along the way was the purchase by the General Services Administration (GSA) in 1985 of 5,000 vehicles equipped with air bags.

Ralph Nader and a group of insurance companies helped convince the GSA chief to purchase vehicles equipped with air bags for the federal government's automotive fleet. With some government subsidies, Ford finally agreed to provide Tempos equipped with air bags. The exemplary safety performance of these air bags provided real-world evidence for the value of government mandating this safety device.

Gerald Carmen, a Republican businessman and the head of GSA at the time, calls the air bag purchase "an exciting adventure, initiated by Nader, supported by the insurance companies, and a real success story for GSA" (quoted in Hemenway 1989, 124).

> LESSON: Government procurement can be used to promote safety
>   and reduce injury.

1.11. Unleaded Gasoline

Lead is a major environmental health hazard to adults, but is even more dangerous to young children. High blood lead levels can result in lowered intelligence (e.g., IQ), learning disabilities, impaired hearing, reduced attention span, hyperactivity, and antisocial behavior. Until the late 1970s, ambient concentrations of lead (from lead that was added to gasoline) were a major contributor to childhood lead poisoning.

In 1972 the Environmental Protection Agency launched an initiative to phase out leaded gasoline; by 1986 the primary phase-out was complete. Average blood levels in children under 6 fell 78 percent between the late 1970s and the early 1990s. The decline was largely due to the phasing out of lead in gasoline; some of the decline was due to legislation banning lead from paint and plumbing supplies. Unfortunately, as of 2008, many developing nations still allowed lead to be added to gasoline.

Getting the lead out of gasoline not only reduced the unintentional injury of childhood lead poisoning, but may also have reduced subsequent intentional violent injuries perpetrated by these children. It is well known that childhood lead exposure can lead to psychological traits that are strongly associated with aggressive and criminal behavior. One controversial study finds that the reduction in lead from gasoline in the late 1970s and early 1980s was responsible for substantial declines in violent crime in the 1990s (Reyes 2007).

Sometimes public health success stories are due to previous public health failures. In 1922 General Motors discovered that adding tetraethyl lead to gasoline raised engine performance by eliminating the "knock." This enhanced the development of the modern automobile. Even then, there was enough awareness of the public health dangers posed that leaded gasoline was banned in New York City for over three years; in 1925 the production of leaded gasoline in the United States was halted for over nine months.

A surgeon general's conference in 1925 brought together the major interested parties in the controversy. As one participant noted, the conference gathered together in one room "two diametrically opposed conceptions. The men engaged in industry—chemists and engineers—take it as a matter of course that a little thing like industrial poisoning should not be allowed to stand in the way of a great industrial advance. On the other hand, the sanitary experts take it as a matter of course that the first consideration is the health of the people" (Rosner & Markowitz 1985, 347).

While Ethyl Corporation claimed that tetraethyl was a "gift of God," the Yale physiologist Yandell Henderson expressed horror that hundreds of thousands of pounds of this slow, cumulative poison would be dispersed in every major city. He accurately foresaw that "conditions would grow worse so gradually and the development of lead poisoning will come on so insidiously . . . that leaded gasoline will be nearly universal . . . before the public and the government will awaken to the situation" (Rosner & Markowitz 1985, 349).

The authorities took the position that they should not act until there was overwhelming evidence that leaded gasoline was actually harming many people. That took another fifty years.

LESSON: Public health may not be the first concern of industry.

1.12. Roundabouts

It is estimated that some 40 percent of all traffic injury collisions in developed countries occur at intersections. Converting intersections from traffic signals to roundabouts, and especially from yield signs to roundabouts, can dramatically reduce injury while increasing traffic flow. Roundabouts have become common at many intersections in the United Kingdom and other European nations.

Roundabouts improve safety in a variety of ways. They reduce the number of conflict points at crossroads from thirty-two to twenty. All traffic comes from one direction in roundabouts, and there are no left turns. Motorists cannot drive a straight path, and thus reduce speed. Finally, motorists entering a roundabout are required to yield to those already in the roundabout and are forced to observe traffic more closely.

At least thirty-three studies have evaluated the effects of roundabouts on traffic safety (Elvik & Vaa 2004). The evidence indicates that changing from yield signs to a roundabout at crossroads reduces injury crashes by about 40 percent; changing from traffic signals to a roundabout reduces injury crashes by approximately 17 percent. Because of the reduction in the speed of the crashing vehicles, the reduction in *serious* injury or fatal crashes may be as high as 70 to 90 percent (Persaud et al. 2001).

In spite of the fact that roundabouts reduce speed, they actually increase mobility, or traffic flow, by eliminating many turning maneuvers and reducing the need to stop. For example, a study from Sweden found that converting an intersection with 23,500 incoming vehicles per day from a traffic light to a roundabout saved motorists an average of 10.1 seconds per car (Varhelyi 1993).

By lowering speed and increasing traffic flow roundabouts also reduce automotive air pollution. For example, a Danish study found that emission of hydrocarbons, carbon monoxide, and nitrogen oxide were about 10 percent lower at roundabouts compared with traffic signals (Bendtsen 1992). A Swedish study found a 29 percent reduction in carbon monoxide emission and a 21 percent reduction in nitrogen oxide emissions after a signalized intersection was converted to a roundabout (Varhelyi 1993).

The conversion of many intersections to roundabouts in Europe has helped reduce traffic injuries while lowering pollution and speeding motorists on their way.

> LESSON: A focus on safety can sometimes lead to improvements in
> other goals, in this case mobility and clean air.

1.13. *Guardrails*

Between 1979 and 1985 twenty-seven fatalities occurred when motorists lost control of their vehicles along the winding roads and plunged over the steep embankments along a hundred-mile stretch of Routes 96, 169, and 299 near the Hoopa, Yurok, and Karok Indian reservations in the vicinity of Willow Creek, California.

In 1985 the California Highway Department installed strong guardrails at fifty sites where the embankments were particularly steep and where fourteen fatalities had occurred in the previous seven years.

In the following ten years, no fatalities were reported at these sites. By contrast, on the rest of this dangerous stretch, the fatality rate did not change; thirteen motorists had died in the previous seven years from going over the embankment, and sixteen died in the subsequent ten years. It is estimated that the guardrails saved two motorists a year from plunging over the embankments and dying.

LESSON: Roads can be made more or less safe.

1.14. Crash Cushions

The vast majority of improvements in roadside safety have occurred since 1960. Prior to that time little attention was given to the roadside; run-off-the-road crashes were attributed to the "nut behind the wheel." This philosophy resulted in untreated guardrail terminals, unyielding signs, and nontraversable ditches. In recent years the general acceptance of the "forgiving roadside" philosophy has helped reduce motor vehicle serious injuries and deaths (Wendling 1996).

Ideally, in a forgiving roadside all roadside hazards would be eliminated and there would be a clear zone so that a vehicle leaving the road would not contact anything. As far as we know, no one has ever died when they lost control of their car and it ran off the road into an open field. While it is often infeasible to eliminate all roadside hazards, the remaining hazards can be made less injurious (e.g., by making lighting columns collapsible). If it is not possible to move the object or make it breakable, the highway authority should provide protection with a safety fence, guard, or barrier.

Crash cushions are energy-absorbing structures installed in front of bridge pillars, tunnel portals, or road dividers at exit ramps. They are designed to safely stop a vehicle within a relatively short distance. Crash cushions do not prevent collisions, but reduce the extent of damage and injury when a collision occurs. Studies from the United States, Great Britain, and the Netherlands indicate that new crash cushions reduce injuries and fatalities in crashes into permanent obstacles by approximately 70 percent (Elvik & Vaa 2004).

Since the early 1960s the use of crash cushions to help protect vehicles from crashes with fixed objects at highway gore areas (e.g., between the exit ramp and the highway) has become a widespread practice in the United States.

LESSON: The built environment can be constructed to reduce the
          seriousness of injury.

HEROES

1.a. Hugh DeHaven (1895–1980)

In World War I, Hugh DeHaven served as a young American volunteer cadet with the Canadian Flying Corps. During combat practice his plane collided with another plane, and both crashed. DeHaven suffered two broken legs and a ruptured liver, pancreas, and gallbladder. The other pilot walked away from his crashed plane.

During his six months of convalescence DeHaven began to consider the features of the aircraft that led to his injuries. He concluded that his own internal injuries were due to the stiff and pointed buckle on his lap belt, which he had jackknifed over at impact, and that solid structures in front of the pilot's head often caused serious injury. When he began to discuss his ideas and findings with his superiors, he encountered resistance and inertia. His commanding officer preferred to attribute escapes from injury to the "Jesus factor" and death to the "luck of the game."

Eighteen years later, a minor automobile crash led DeHaven to recall his earlier ideas about vehicle structure and unintentional injury. He presented his ideas to a special committee for aviation medicine and other groups. He again found little or no interest in improving survivability; the argument was that money would be better used if spent to prevent the accident from occurring in the first place (the pre-event).

Between 1938 and 1941 DeHaven personally investigated aircraft crashes and falls from heights. In 1942 he published his seminal paper on surviving falls, and he was appointed director of a project called Crash Injury Research at Cornell University Medical College.

DeHaven's 1942 article presents case studies of eight falls from heights, falls that could well have led to death but in which the people not only survived, but had little serious injury. For example, in Case 1 a 42-year-old woman jumped from the sixth floor and fell onto fairly well-packed earth in a garden plot, landing on her left side and back. The superintendent of the building reached the victim immediately after she struck the ground. She raised herself on her left elbow and remarked, "Six stories and not hurt." Later in life DeHaven said that these eight cases "did more to support [his] theories about crash injuries and crash survival than all the words in the dictionary," and that at the time the article was written, "people knew more about protecting eggs in transit than they did about protecting human heads."

DeHaven's work provided strong evidence that the human body was less fragile than had generally been assumed, that the structural environment was the dominant cause of injury, and that the environment could be modified to reduce the likelihood of injury. He argued that the basic laws of physics operated for human injuries, and the distribution of force largely determines the damage inflicted. His analyses formed the basis for many of the most effective injury prevention measures used today, including soft playground surfaces, air bags, and helmets.

DeHaven is considered a genuine pioneer. Although hundreds of combat pilots had died as a result of injuries sustained in crashing, DeHaven seems to have been the first to seriously give consideration to the actual cause of death. The same held true for car crash victims. Automobile manufacturers did not have the type of safety departments they have today, and there was little basic scientific research. Much of the early fundamental work in crash protection was due to the efforts of DeHaven, who for years financed his own research in this new area.

DeHaven's work at Cornell was aimed at reducing the direct cause of airplane and motor vehicle injuries: the secondary impact between the occupant and the interior of the vehicle. For example, by the early 1950s DeHaven and his associates had conceived, designed, and tested almost all of the features that would later be incorporated into automobile safety belts. His work demonstrated that human bodies could withstand forces of severe car crashes without death or serious injury if they were properly "packaged." DeHaven is sometimes called the father of crashworthiness research.

Later in life, DeHaven received numerous awards, and his status in the injury field is now high. However, virtually no one outside the automotive and aviation safety field knows his name. As of August 2008 his name did not appear in Wikipedia.

1.b. John Paul Stapp (1910–1999)

John Paul Stapp, a physician, PhD, and Air Force colonel, became famous as "the fastest man on earth," traveling faster than a speeding bullet. He also was the fastest man to stop (decelerate). His scientific work helped reduce the risk for aviators, and his advocacy helped save the lives of many motorists.

In the early 1940s Stapp began studying the effects of high-altitude flights on pilots, particularly how they could prevent dehydration, freezing, and the bends (the deadly formation of bubbles in the blood). The final problem was the most difficult, but after many flights in subzero temperatures, Stapp discovered the answer: if a pilot breathed pure oxygen for thirty minutes prior to takeoff, symptoms could be avoided.

After this success Stapp was assigned the problem of human deceleration, the body's ability to withstand G forces (a G is defined as the force of gravity acting on a human on Earth at sea level). At the time, 18Gs was considered the most a human could expect to survive; as a result, military cockpits were built to withstand only an 18G impact.

Stapp not only supervised experiments on the rocket sled track, but he was his own test subject. He suffered concussions, lost dental fillings, and found that for G forces, the most vulnerable part of the human anatomy was the eye. He also showed the inadequacy of certain Air Force restraint systems and that rearward-facing occupants could survive higher G loads than forward-facing ones. Most important, he debunked the 18G limit. If humans could tolerate 30G decelerations, seat belts and cockpits needed to be built so that pilots could survive such a deceleration.

With aircraft beginning to travel at supersonic speed, the next issue was whether pilots could survive ejection at such speeds. On December 10, 1954, on a test track in New Mexico, Stapp strapped himself in for his twenty-ninth (and final) sled ride. In five seconds he was accelerated to 632 mph, then brought to a complete halt—in 1.4 seconds.

For more than a second, Stapp endured 25Gs, the equivalent of a Mach 1.6 ejection at 40,000 feet (a force about the same as crashing into a wall at 120 mph). He suffered complete red out, as nearly every capillary in his eyeballs burst. Fortunately, by the next day, his eyesight had returned.

Stapp became an instant celebrity. He was labeled not only the fastest man on earth but also "the bravest man in the Air Force." He was featured on the covers of *Life* and *Collier's* magazines, and became the subject of a Hollywood movie. He used his fame to promote the cause of automotive safety.

Stapp persuaded the Air Force to build an automotive testing facility, and he conducted the first-ever crash tests with dummies. He also convinced the Air Force to take up the automotive safety cause by providing statistics showing that more Air Force pilots were killed in traffic accidents than in plane crashes.

At every opportunity Stapp lobbied for the installation of seat belts (not even an option on most 1954 cars), soft dashboards, collapsible steering columns, and shock-absorbing bumpers. "I'm leading a crusade for the prevention of needless deaths," he told *Time* magazine, making its cover in 1955.

In 1966, when President Lyndon Johnson signed a law requiring seat belts in all new cars, Stapp was by his side. "The fastest man on earth" received numerous awards before his death, including the Presidential Medal of Technology and the Legion of Merit.

1.c. William Haddon Jr. (1926–1985)

Bill Haddon is probably the best known of all injury control professionals. The Haddon matrix is one of the first concepts taught in every injury prevention course. A tool to help systematically identify all options available to reduce injuries, the Haddon matrix divides possible interventions into three phases (pre-event, event, postevent) and three factors (human, agent, environment).

During the first sixty years of motor vehicle use, research and prevention efforts were focused almost exclusively at the pre-event, human factor: the bad driver. It was claimed that over 90 percent of crashes were due to driver error, so naturally the goal became to improve the driver. Yet education and enforcement efforts were not always successful at changing driver behavior or reducing injuries. Haddon helped change this exclusive focus on the driver to one that included the vehicle and the road.

"It is hard to overemphasize the importance . . . of the conceptual shift from this single-cause, behavioral explanations of injury to multiple-cause, environmental explanations" (Christoffel & Gallagher 1999, 32). With many possible countermeasures, the choice became picking the most cost-effective ones. These were often changes to the agent (e.g., the motor vehicle) or the environment (e.g., the highway), rather than attempts to change human nature. And the most successful interventions were often "passive" measures (a word coined by Haddon), measures that protected the individual automatically, without any action on his or her part (e.g., collapsible steering columns, air bags).

Most traffic safety interventions in the 1950s were based on "expert opinion"; there was little good scientific information to back them up. High school driver education classes, for example, have long been popular, though we know today that they do not reduce crashes or save lives. However, many states allow teenagers who take these classes to drive at a younger age, when they are at high risk for injury (Robertson 1998). Haddon insisted that the injury field be based less on opinion and more on science. At traffic safety meetings, when supposed experts made assertions, Haddon was known to ask, "Where are the studies?"

Usually there were no scientific studies, and often the assertion was wrong.

Haddon himself undertook many of the early scientific studies in injury prevention. He and his colleagues, for example, were the first to document the large role played by alcohol in fatal highway crashes and pedestrian fatalities (ICADTS Reporter 1999). He also contributed substantially to the methodology of the injury field. For example, some motorists are likely to have more crashes simply because they drive more, on more dangerous streets, or at more dangerous times. Unfortunately there are rarely good data available on such measures of "exposure." Haddon and his colleagues developed a method to control for exposure when it was not possible to actually measure the amount of exposure. For injuries occurring in public settings, Haddon's method was to compare the motorist in a crash to a control population of uninjured persons at the site of the injury event at the same time of day and day of the week.

Haddon was versed in epidemiology, medicine, and engineering. He received his undergraduate degree from MIT and his medical and public health degrees from Harvard. But Haddon was more than a scientist. He also directed major institutions that made important changes. As Ralph Nader said of Haddon, "He connected knowledge to action in the great tradition of preventive medicine. His was a rare combination of being a thinker and a doer" (ICADTS Reporter 1999, 3). As the Johns Hopkins University injury expert Sue Baker (1997, 371) noted, "Haddon set a great example to all of us in passionately fighting to have public policy based on fact rather than myth and guesswork, and to have regulations shaped by public need rather than private profit."

In 1966 Haddon became the first administrator of the National Highway Safety Bureau (now the National Highway Traffic Safety Administration). During his tenure the agency issued the first safety requirements for new vehicles, including requirements for shoulder belts, laminated windshields, energy-absorbing steering columns, and side door beams. Later, almost identical vehicle standards were adopted in Canada, Australia, and a number of countries in Europe (O'Neill 2002). From 1969 to his death in 1985 he served as the president of the Insurance Institute for Highway Safety. With Haddon at the helm, this nonprofit institution, supported entirely by automobile insurance companies, became an internationally known research organization and joined the effort to transform the highway safety field. The institute continues to be a leader in providing unbiased information on motor vehicle safety. Other areas of injury prevention lack such a strong insurance voice. More than anyone else, Bill Haddon "produced or strongly influenced the thinking that is central to understanding of the field" of injury prevention (Robertson 1983, 71).

The contributions of DeHaven, Stapp, Haddon, and others were successful in shifting injury prevention "away from an early, naive preoccupation with distributing educational pamphlets and posters and toward modifying the environments in which injuries occur" (National Committee for Injury Prevention and Control 1989, 7).

1.d. Ralph Nader (1934–)

As a law student at Harvard, Ralph Nader published an article in *The Nation* in 1959 entitled "The Safe Car You Can't Buy." He elaborated on this theme in his 1965 book, *Unsafe at Any Speed: The Designed-in Dangers of the American Automobile.* Using the sporty Corvair as an illustration, the book documented how Detroit subordinated safety to styling.

Although sales of the book were initially modest, General Motors' concern about litigation regarding the Corvair's safety led it to hire private detectives to tail Nader to dig up information that might discredit him. The story broke in the *New Republic,* and Connecticut Senator Abraham Ribicoff's subcommittee (to which Nader had acted as an unpaid advisor) summoned the president of GM, who was forced to apologize publicly to Nader.

This remarkable incident catapulted automobile safety, and Nader, into the public spotlight and sent his book to the top of the best-seller list. Senate hearings in 1966 led to the creation of a new federal agency, the forerunner of the National Highway Traffic Safety Administration, with power to create safety performance standards, conduct investigations, and order recalls. In 1977 Henry Ford conceded on *Meet the Press,* "We wouldn't have the kinds of safety built into automobiles that we have had unless there had been a federal law."

The GM incident ratified a core Nader conviction: that a few people, acting with truth and persistence, could make a difference. Nader was not a one-issue wonder, but built his fame into the largest consumer and citizen movement in American history. Real patriotism, he claimed, was caring enough about your country to get involved and do something to make it more moral and caring. Instead of being an inconsequential private citizen, one should become an engaged "public citizen."

In the late 1960s Nader's advocacy in the injury area helped create federal standards for the safety of natural gas pipelines and radiation limits for microwave ovens, sun lamps, and televisions. Injury prevention, however, has been only one small part of Nader's work to improve society. He has "dedicated his life to good citizenship and showing others how to put democracy into action" (Marcello 2004, xi).

1.e. Seymour Charles (1921–2002) and Robert Sanders (1927–2006)

During one Thanksgiving weekend in the early 1960s a young patient of the pediatrician Seymour Charles was killed in an automobile crash. The child, who had not been restrained by any safety device, had flown through the car window and died instantly. That incident transformed Dr. Charles into a crusader for automobile safety.

After the death Charles attended an automobile safety conference held in Detroit. At the meeting he stood and asked why the engineers were not designing cars to protect the occupants. With the encouragement of Ralph Nader, Charles (with Annemarie Shelness) organized Physicians for Automotive Safety (PAS). In 1965 the group picketed outside the Coliseum in New York City, where automakers were holding their annual new car show. Charles remained the PAS president until it closed shop in 1989.

In the 1960s Charles testified before Congress about car safety and was invited to the White House Rose Garden when President Lyndon Johnson signed the legislation creating the Department of Transportation. Before he died in 2002 Charles received a citation from the American Academy of Pediatrics as the "leading national advocate for child auto safety."

In 1975 Charles's article in the journal *Pediatrics* on children in cars served as a wake-up call for pediatricians and advocates nationwide. That article, and the work of PAS, inspired a Tennessee pediatrician, Robert Sanders, and his wife, Pat, to press for the passage of a state mandatory child restraint law, which was enacted in 1978. By 1985 all fifty states had enacted similar laws.

Sanders headed a Tennessee county health department for over twenty years. A soft-spoken physician, he proved to be a tough, persuasive lobbyist. He believed that car seats were like vaccines in preventing death and injury in highway crashes. A tireless fighter for passenger safety generally, he became known as "Dr. Seatbelt."

In 2006 the Robert Sanders Award was created for Outstanding Public Policy Achievement in Child Passenger Safety. At the ceremony, the General Motors director of auto safety said, "Dr. Sanders was a true pioneer whose legacy is improved safety for generations of the nation's most precious cargo—our children."

1.f. Candy Lightner (1946–)

In 1980 a drunk hit-and-run driver killed Candy Lightner's 13-year-old daughter, Cari, while she was walking in a bicycle lane on her way to a church carnival in suburban Sacramento, California. The driver had four prior arrests for drunk driving; one had occurred two days before the tragedy. For killing Cari he served no jail time, only nine months at a work camp and halfway house. Outraged, Lightner and a group of friends decided to form an organization to lobby for stiffer penalties for drunk drivers. They called their organization Mothers Against Drunk Drivers, or MADD.

Lightner previously was "neither registered to vote, nor able to distinguish Democrat from Republican" (Frantzich 2005, 80), but she quickly became a political force. She sat through court hearings and watched the lenient way the judicial system typically handled drunk driving cases. "One judge said to me: 'If you don't like the law little lady, go and change it,' and I said: 'O.K., I will'" (Creamer 1984). She established a mailing list of parents who had also lost their children to drunk drivers and called for the creation of task forces at all levels of government— local, state, and federal—to investigate the problem.

Lightner asked President Ronald Reagan to create a commission on drunk driving and gathered a hundred people to picket the White House when he didn't respond. This event received such news coverage that California governor Jerry Brown, who had previously been unwilling to meet with her, not only met her but established a governor's task force on the issue. In 1982 President Reagan created a National Commission against Drunk Driving and appointed Lightner to serve on the board of directors.

Through lectures, speeches, published works, and personal appearances Lightner helped create a movement. Only two years after its creation, a national survey found that 84 percent of the U.S. population had heard about MADD. In 1983 NBC produced a television movie about Lightner, and the *Ladies' Home Journal* named her one of the top one hundred women in America.

In 1983 the government reported that 129 new anti–drunk driving laws had been passed that year, and in 1984 President Reagan signed a law raising the federal minimum drinking age to 21. When Lightner left MADD in 1985 it had over 350 local chapters and more than half a million members and donors.

MADD helped to create a sea change in American attitudes and policies concerning drunk driving. The organization works to pass strong anti–drunk driver laws; to ensure strong enforcement of these laws, its volunteers attend drunk driving court cases and report the outcome to the media. MADD deserves much of the credit for the reduction in alcohol-related traffic fatalities in the United States. Between 1982 and 2000 these declined 34 percent, and the percentage of the nation's traffic fatalities that were alcohol-related fell from 60 to 41 (National Highway Traffic Safety Administration 2002).

CHAPTER 2

Home

INTRODUCTION

The rate of injury in the home is highest for children and the elderly. The elderly are at increased risk because they have reduced vision and balance and are generally more frail than younger adults. Children lack the physical and cognitive abilities of adults and thus need more protection.

The American Medical Association provides recommendations for preventing many common household accidents. "Life can't be risk-free," they advise, "but most household accidents can be prevented by using a household safety checklist. This will help you identify and eliminate potential hazards in your home." Examples of advice include "Never leave infants under one year old alone with a family pet"; "Don't drink hot beverages or soup with a child sitting on your lap"; "Don't leave children unattended by a pool, wading pool, or hot tub—even for a moment"; "Cover all unused outlets with safety caps"; and "Keep side rails up on cribs" (American Medical Association 2005).

The success stories in this section all come from the post–World War II era and include the prevention of poisoning (child-resistant packaging), electrocutions (hair dryers), burns and scalds (smoke detectors, flammability of pajamas, tap water burns, burns from cigarette lighters), falls (window guards), and crushing (wringer arm). Most of these successes deal with reducing injuries to children, and most focus on the pre-event. They provide examples of successes in making the home environment safe for children, rather than simply trying to educate the child about possible dangers. Children are not little adults; they need protection. "A house is an exciting place for infants and small children, who love to explore but aren't aware of the potential dangers. Protecting your child from household dangers is your job—and it's a job that will always be evolving to keep up with your child's growing mobility and curiosity" (American Medical Association 2005).

Many voluntary and mandatory product standards have been created to reduce the risk of injury. For example, minimum dimensions of rattles and pacifiers and reduced spacing for crib slats are mandated to reduce the risk of asphyxiation (Baker & Fisher 1980).

Changes in technology and fashion can have positive or negative effects on safety. Benefits in the twentieth century include the reduction in kerosene poisoning caused by rural electrification. The replacement of coal home heating by oil and natural gas dramatically reduced carbon monoxide poisoning in the United States. Serious clothing burns to girls fell substantially when pants replaced loose-fitting dresses as the fashion, and improvements in washing machines effectively eliminated "wringer arm." New products can also create new dangers. One of the success stories deals with actions to prevent a new product, infant walkers, from injuring children.

Protecting your child is one of the most important personal responsibilities in life. But it is difficult for parents to go it alone. It is helpful to have supportive relatives and friends and live in a society that reduces the temptations and dangers to which children are exposed. The stories in this chapter are of policies that have successfully helped parents protect their children against serious injury.

HOME SUCCESS STORIES

2.1. Child-Resistant Packaging

In the 1960s more than 11,000 young children were poisoned each year from accidental overdoses of baby aspirin. The Poison Prevention Packaging Act of 1970 required that aspirin be packaged in child-resistant closures. In anticipation of the law, by 1970 the two largest manufacturers of baby aspirin had introduced safety closures. Comparing the three years prior to these changes (1967–1969) to the three years after (1971–1973), baby aspirin poisoning of children under 5 years fell more than 70 percent.

Since then, improved medical care, warning labels, the reduction in the number of tablets per bottle, and the decrease in baby aspirin use due to its connection with Reye's syndrome have further reduced the number of young children accidentally dying from overdoses of aspirin. In 1960 in the United States, 144 young children died from accidental overdoses of aspirin. By 1988 that number had fallen to 3.

In addition to baby aspirin, the Poisoning Prevention Packaging Act required child-resistant packaging for a variety of products (e.g., antifreeze, drain cleaners, oven cleaners, lighter fluid), but not others (e.g., laundry soaps and detergents, cosmetics, alcoholic beverages, and numerous household chemicals). Nationally between 1973 and 1978, while child-poisoning rates from the unregulated products remained constant, rates from the newly regulated products fell by 67 percent (Walton 1982).

> LESSON: It is possible to protect children without changing their or
>   their parents' behavior.

2.2. Hair Dryer Electrocutions

In the United States in the early 1980s handheld hair dryers caused an average of eighteen electrocution deaths per year; most of the victims were in bathtubs, and children were at greatest risk. Government (the Consumer Product Safety Commission [CPSC]), industry, and voluntary standards organizations (Underwriters' Laboratories [UL]) worked together to prevent these tragedies. In 1980 the UL standard began requiring a pictorial warning against the use of hair dryers in bathtubs. In 1987 the standard required that new hair dryers provide protection against electrocutions when the product was immersed in water and the switch was off. In 1991 UL-certified handheld hair dryers required protection in the "on" as well as the "off" position. The CPSC and manufacturer research and technology were key in enabling such improvements. The number of electrocutions associated with hair dryers fell to four per year in the early 1990s; by 2000 there was only one such death.

> LESSON: Government, industry, and voluntary standards
>   organizations can work together to reduce injury.

2.3. Residential Smoke Detectors

The most dangerous residential fires occur at night, when most people are asleep. Smoke detectors help protect the family by providing early warning of fire. It is estimated that a working smoke detector reduces the risk of residential fire death by almost 50 percent.

In 1969 Randolph Smith and Kenneth House patented the first
battery-powered smoke detector. Smoke alarms rapidly became a
familiar presence in American homes. Homes with smoke detectors
increased from 5 percent in 1970 to 75 percent in 1985 to nearly 94
percent in 2000. The key factor in this increase was the low price of
these battery-powered alarms. In the early 1970s the cost of protecting a three-bedroom home with professionally installed alarms was
approximately $1,000. By the mid-1990s the cost of owner-installed
alarms in the same house had fallen to $10 per alarm, or less than $50
for the entire house.

Other factors, such as marketing campaigns, building code modifications, and legislation requiring detectors in homes, were also important.
By the mid-1980s, for example, laws requiring that smoke alarms be
placed in all new and existing residences existed in thirty-eight states
and thousands of municipalities. The increase in smoke detectors is generally credited with being an important reason why the residential fire
fatality rate fell from approximately 2.4 deaths per 100,000 people in
1970 to 1.0 death per 100,000 in 2000. The National Fire Protection
Association says that "smoke alarms are the residential fire safety success story of the past quarter century" (National Fire Protection
Association 2008).

A current concern is that many battery-powered alarms in homes
don't work. Another problem is that some of the very poor may still not
have detectors. The importance of detectors is illustrated by the highly
successful community intervention that occurred in an area of
Oklahoma City in 1990. Although that area included only 16 percent of
the city population, from 1987 to 1990 it experienced 45 percent of the
city's total residential fire injuries and death, a fire injury rate four times
higher than the rest of the city population. During that period, only four
of the thirty fire fatalities and injuries in this area occurred in homes
with functioning smoke detectors. The intervention consisted of giving
out and testing smoke alarms as well as providing educational materials
to households. Over the next six years (1990–1996) the fire injury rate
fell 81 percent in the intervention community; by comparison, it fell
only 7 percent in the rest of the city (Mallonee 2000). It is estimated
that in the first five years postintervention the program prevented twenty
fatal and twenty-four nonfatal fire injuries (Haddix et al. 2001).

LESSON: Technological innovations leading to improved
performance and lower price are often crucial in reducing
injury.

2.4. Flammability of Children's Pajamas

Flame burns are among the most serious and painful of injuries. In the early 1970s the Consumer Product Safety Commission adopted two federal standards regarding the flammability of children's sleepwear. Although national data are not available to evaluate the effect of the law, data from the Shriners Pediatric Burn Institute in Boston showed that the rate of pajama burns fell from twelve children per year in the five years before the standards (1969–1973) to two children per year for two years after the standard (1975–1976). There was no trend evident in referrals for burns because of ignition of clothing other than sleepwear.

Similarly, data from the Shriners Pediatric Burn Unit in Galveston showed a decrease in sleepwear-related injuries from eleven per year (1966–1973) to fewer than four per year (1974–1977). There was no significant change in admissions due to ignition of other clothing; sleepwear-related injuries as a percentage of total burn cases dropped significantly. In most of the pajama burn cases after the law was enacted, the victim was wearing hand-me-down articles manufactured prior to the promulgation of the standards.

LESSON: Product changes are often the most cost-effective way of reducing injury.

2.5. Tap Water Burns

Ordinary household tap water can be a major source of injury. The typical hot water temperature found in Canadian homes in the late 1990s was 140 degrees Fahrenheit. Exposed to water at this temperature, a young child's skin will be severely burned in less than five seconds. Tap water scalds tend to be the most severe form of scalding injuries among children. For example, in the late 1990s at the Hospital for Sick Children in Toronto, children scalded by hot tap water were hospitalized for approximately twenty-three days, while the average length of stay for children scalded by other means was ten days.

The United States has made better progress than Canada in reducing the tap water injury problem. In the 1970s water heater industry practice was to factory-preset water heaters at 140 to 150 degrees. In 1977 Seattle homes had a mean hot water temperature of 142 degrees. In 1983 a Washington state law required that all new water heaters be preset at 120 degrees. In 1988 the mean hot water temperature in Seattle homes had fallen to 122 degrees. Burn admission rates for King County (Seattle) children (under age 15) for tap water scalds fell dramatically, from 5.5 per year in 1969–1976 to 2.3 per year in 1984–1988. Most of the burns in the latter period were due to child abuse rather than accidents.

All new electric heaters in the United States are preset at 120 degrees and are shipped with appropriate warning labels. Still, in 2000 the heaters were set at a higher temperature when exported to Canada. In the late 1990s it was estimated that more than five hundred Canadian children were hospitalized each year due to hot tap water burns.

> LESSON: Passive safety measures can effectively reduce severe
> injuries to children.

2.6. Wringer Arm

The term "wringer arm" was introduced in a 1938 *New England Journal of Medicine* article that described more than two dozen cases of children injured when their arm was drawn between the rollers of a wringer-type clothes washer. Over the next thirty-five years more than twenty-five medical articles were written concerning the incidence and treatment of these injuries. One study, for example, analyzed more than 450 patients treated in a three-year period (1965–1968) at the hand surgical service of Cook County Hospital in Chicago; 180 of the patients were between the ages of 3 and 5. Over one-sixth of the patients required operative procedures.

In 1968 Underwriters' Laboratories certification began requiring that all new wringer washers have either a "dead man switch" or an "instinctive release" to stop the roller when meeting a twenty-pound force. More important, by the early 1960s sales of spin-dry washers were surpassing those of wringer washing machines. By 1970 wringer machines accounted for only 5 percent of sales of new machines; production of wringer washers ceased in the United States in 1983. Automatic spin-dry machines are much safer; in the decade of the 1990s, although wringer machines represented only a small percentage of all operating washing machines, they accounted for almost half of all incidents in which a washing machine was the primary cause of an injury. Virtually all of the wringer injuries occurred to the arm; many were caused when a finger or hand was caught in clothing and the arm pulled through the ringers.

Automatic spin-dry washing machines include locking lid mechanisms and tubs that automatically stop agitating when the lid is open. Although these mechanisms could be improved, serious washing machine injuries have fallen dramatically; wringer arm is disappearing from American life. Most primary automatic spin-dry washing machine injuries now occur when the victim is hit by a falling lid or deliberately places a body part into the running water. The large majority of secondary washing machine injuries involve children falling from or jumping from the washer or people knocking into the machine. Safety experts now urge parents not to put children in car or baby seats on top of operating machines.

LESSON: Technology can both create and alleviate injury problems.

2.7. Infant Walkers

Many parents believe that walkers not only provide entertainment for young children but also help teach them to walk. Walkers do keep the child occupied so the parent can attend to other things. Unfortunately studies show that these walkers actually delay normal motor and mental development, and the enhanced mobility allows the child to get into dangerous situations: gaining access to oven doors, heavy objects, poisonous substances, and staircases. In the 1990s the large majority of injuries related to infant walkers were head injuries caused by falling down stairs.

In the 1980s and early 1990s a number of active intervention strategies were employed to reduce the danger. These included public awareness campaigns, physician advice to parents ("anticipatory guidance"), and warning labels (advising adult supervision during walker use and use of barriers such as stair gates). These active strategies, which require human vigilance, appeared to have little effect on child safety: the number of walker-related injuries to infants (most 7 to 10 months old) that required emergency department visits remained at over 20,000 per year, with some 1,000 requiring hospitalization.

In the early 1990s the American Academy of Pediatrics and the American Medical Association called for a ban on the sale of mobile baby walkers. This did not happen, but in the mid-1990s the U.S. Consumer Product Safety Commission worked with industry to create two passive prevention strategies (passive strategies provide automatic protection, without any action on the part of the caregiver or child). The American Society for Testing and Materials (ASTM), an institution organized for the development of voluntary standards, arrived at by consensus, with strict guidelines for due process and balanced committee membership, revised their existing voluntary performance standard for infant walkers. The goal was to reduce the likelihood of stairway falls: the base of the walker had to be too wide to fit through the standard doorway, and the walker had to incorporate a feature to stop the walker at the edge of a step. At about the same time, stationary activity centers were introduced into the market as an alternative to mobile infant walkers. Stationary walkers do not have wheels.

Injuries to infants from walkers fell dramatically. In 1994 an estimated 23,300 injuries occurred; by 2001 that number had fallen to 5,100—a 76 percent decrease. The decrease was primarily for injuries caused by stairway falls. Most of the injuries in 2001 involved older mobile units that did not meet the revised ASTM standard. In 2004 Canada (but not the United States) banned infant walkers.

> LESSON: The best injury prevention strategies are usually those that
> do not require frequent human action and vigilance.

2.8. Child Window Falls

Window falls of children are a serious urban public health problem. For example, in a five-year period in the late 1960s in New York City, over 120 children 14 years old and younger died after falling from a window. In 1972 the city's Health Department initiated an education and prevention program called Children Can't Fly in a high-risk area of the Bronx. The education program included spots on radio and TV and news stories; in addition, over 16,000 free (costing the city $3 each), easy-to-install window guards were distributed to families with preschool-age children living in tenements. Reported falls in the Bronx fell 50 percent in two years. There were no falls reported from windows where guards had been installed.

The New York City Health Department mandated that by 1979 all owners of multiple dwellings in the city had to provide window guards in apartments where children under 11 years old resided. Harlem Hospital records showed a 94 percent decline in accidental falls from windows by children in 1979–1981 compared to 1970–1978: from an average of sixteen every three years to one every three years.

> LESSON: Society can successfully help parents protect their children.

2.9 Child-Resistant Cigarette Lighters

It is estimated that in the United States in the late 1980s children younger than 5 playing with disposable cigarette lighters set more than 5,000 fires annually, leading to over 1,000 injuries. The Consumer

Product Safety Commission worked with a leading voluntary standards group, the American Society for Testing and Materials, to develop a voluntary standard for a child-resistant disposable cigarette lighter. Several manufacturers provided child-resistant designs, enabling the CPSC to establish that the standard was technically feasible. During the development of the voluntary standard, a number of states (e.g., California, Connecticut, New Jersey) either passed or were considering legislation to require child-resistant lighters.

The Lighter Association Inc., representing the manufacturers and importers of lighters, asked the CPSC to adopt the draft ASTM voluntary standard as a mandatory standard. The industry wanted a mandatory standard to preempt potentially conflicting state requirements and to level the playing field. A mandatory standard would ensure that all domestic and foreign manufacturers would be forced to meet the same requirements. The standard went into effect in 1994.

A study by CPSC indicated that, comparing the late 1980s with the late 1990s, fires started by young children playing with cigarette lighters fell 58 percent. Annually, this represents some three thousand fewer fires and six hundred fewer injuries.

Canada adopted a similar standard in 1994. In Australia between 1994 and 1997 the deaths of nine children were directly blamed on non-child-resistant cigarette lighters. Australia adopted a mandatory lighter standard in 1997, and New Zealand followed suit. Beginning in 2007 the European Union required all member states to ensure that cigarette lighters were child-resistant when placed on the EU market.

LESSON: Public health successes in one region are often picked up
          by other locales, saving more lives.

HEROES

2.a. Jay Arena (1909–1995)

In May 1948 two children, ages 2 and 4, were admitted to Duke Hospital in Durham, North Carolina. Each had eaten an entire bottle of the new St. Joseph's flavored aspirin for children, as if the pills were candy. Both died. Nationwide, some two hundred children per year were dying from ingesting aspirin.

Abe Plough was the head of a small pharmaceutical company in Memphis. Their big seller was St. Joseph's aspirin for adults. In the late 1940s they developed a children's line—pink-colored, flavored, and half the dose of the adult aspirin. Put in bottles of one hundred and popularly known as "candy aspirin," the aspirin was a commercial success.

After the second child died, Jay Arena, a Duke pediatrician, picked up the phone and called Mr. Plough. Dr. Arena said, "Look, we've had two children die here at Duke from your product. I think it's a fine product, but I think it's a dangerous product. And you have to do something about it." Plough said, "Yeah, we have been hearing some rumors about that." Arena shouted, "It's more than just rumors!" and repeated that Plough should do something. "Like what, Doctor?" Arena hadn't given it much thought. He said off the top of his head, "It seems to me you could develop something to make it very difficult for a child to get to these candy aspirin. . . . How about a different top?"

Plough sent over one of his vice presidents to talk with Arena; they decided to work together. First the drug company did some research and came to Arena with seventeen possible closures. Arena tested these with the families of his young patients in Durham and picked the one that worked the best.

Over twenty years before the Poison Prevention Packaging Act made such closures mandatory, Plough decided to put this safety closure on his St. Joseph's aspirin. But no other company would do the same thing. The day before he was scheduled to put the closure on the market, he called Arena and said, "I'm literally scared to death about what we're doing. And I am tempted to withdraw from this. . . . I think I'll lose sales, and I think our little company will go down the drain." Arena said, "You know that if you present the reason for your use of the safety closure before the public, tell them why you are doing it, I don't think you're going to lose sales. I think you might gain sales." There was a long silence over the phone. Arena says he will remember that as long as he lives. He thought, "He's not going to do it. He's not going to do it. He's just scared to death." Then Plough said, "Dr. Arena, if it saves the life of one child, I'll do it."

Sales of St. Joseph's children's aspirin increased the next year by 25 percent.

Over the years Arena worked with Plough to cut down the number of tablets per bottle to fifty, and then to thirty-six. The dose was also cut down by one half, so even if a 2-year-old child ate the entire bottle, the dose would not be toxic. That's what every company does now—by law.

Says Arena, "Of all the things I've done and accomplished, I'm more proud of that than anything because I know from personal experience, and I know from the experience of hundreds, thousands of my colleagues, that this safety closure has saved children's lives. Not just from aspirin, but from drugs. Now the law makes it mandatory to put safety packaging [on] dangerous household products like Drano, furniture polish and many other products." And the public can have their medication without a safety closure simply by asking the pharmacist.

Dr. Arena has reason to be proud of other accomplishments. In the 1930s childhood poisoning was a significant component of pediatric practice, but little information existed about the ingredients or the toxicity of many products, or the best treatments. Arena began keeping reference files on all types of poisoning. The file eventually led to an inventory of products and treatments for poisoning and helped to develop the Duke Poison Control Center and more than six hundred other poison control centers across the United States.

In the 1930s, when a child ingested a household product there was usually nothing labeled to tell the physician what it contained. If a child did not respond to treatment, Arena would personally call the medical director of the company. Sometimes the company would provide the ingredients, and sometimes not; often they would say, "It's a trade secret." Arena would say, "This child might die, and if this child dies, the press is going to know about it. He died from your product. And that you wouldn't give us the information." If that didn't work, Arena would call the president of the company. And he would get the information.

In those days the industry was not terribly cooperative. Arena comments, "But you can't say that now. They have been great. They know that they have an important role in the prevention of these poisoning accidents. . . . I think it's a different ballgame."

2.b. Bent Sorensen (1924–)

Dr. Bent Sorensen, a surgeon in the Department of Plastic Surgery, created the Burns Unit at the University of Copenhagen. He classified burn prevention into major and minor prevention. Major prevention requires changing the culture, or way of life. For example, he cited burn dangers caused by native garments that easily catch fire, such as saris worn by women in India who originally prepared meals over an open-air fire and continued to do so over Primus stoves, indoors in small apartments, and the voluminous costumes worn by Algerian women that were suitable for life in the desert but dangerous in small dwellings. Minor prevention included those initiatives that require only changes in habits or regulations.

Sorensen was instrumental in inducing many types of minor prevention that led to reduced injuries from burns and scalds.

In 1971 the people of Denmark consumed approximately 7 billion cups of coffee; some three thousand Danes had to be treated that year for scalds due to coffee. Using data from the Copenhagen Burns Unit, Sorenson and a colleague found that close to 60 percent of the scalds were caused by the coffee filter tipping over. Their 1973 paper highlighted this fact and was widely cited in newspapers and magazines and on television. Sorenson's advice was to throw away the wobbly filters and acquire a more stable type, or at least to brew coffee in the kitchen sink rather than on the kitchen table. The factory producing the filters agreed to produce the new type (but would not withdraw the old filter from the market). The combination of product change and education worked. Data from the Burns Unit showed that, compared to 1971, in 1973–1974, coffee scalds in Denmark fell 67 percent.

In the early 1970s Sorensen performed plastic surgery on a severely scalded child who had been burned at a self-service laundry. The burns occurred when the child opened the door of a washing machine that was filling with very hot water (176 degrees Fahrenheit). To allow consecutive wash cycles to start with a minimum of delay between customers, the water temperature in these laundries was set much higher than in home washing machines. Sorenson discovered that about three young children each year in Copenhagen were being severely scalded in such incidents. He contacted the government's Labor Inspection Service, which issued a regulation on September 1, 1971, requiring that special safety locks be installed on the doors of front-loading washing machines if water of more than 120 degrees could rise above the lower rim of the gate. Over the next three years there were no cases of this type of scald; the problem was solved.

These are just two instances of Sorenson's actions to promote the public's health. They provide "outstanding examples of how a physician can function as a community injury-prevention advocate" (Berger & Mohan 1996, 183).

2.c. Ken Feldman (1944–) and Murray Katcher (1945–)

Seattle pediatrician Ken Feldman's experience with scald burns among his patients led him to question why such seemingly preventable injuries occurred. He analyzed hospital data to determine the extent of the problem and the circumstances of the injury. Tap water scald burns were often more severe and disabling and more extensive and required longer hospitalization than other types of scald burns. At high risk were children under age 5.

With his wife, Ann, and a community health aide from his clinic, Feldman knocked on doors and measured the tap water temperatures in homes and apartments in the surrounding area. They found that the mean bathtub water temperature was 142 degrees (full-thickness burns can occur in adult skin in two seconds at 150 degrees). In Seattle at the time, gas water heaters were preset at 140 degrees (six seconds for a full-thickness scald of adult skin) and electric heaters at 150 degrees; the power companies recommended water temperatures at 140 to 150 degrees. Feldman reported all this in 1978 in the lead article in the journal *Pediatrics*.

The easiest way to prevent these injuries was clear: lower the temperature of the water by changing the preset temperature of the water heater. Although his petition to the Consumer Product Safety Commission was unsuccessful, Feldman led a somewhat more successful educational campaign, in conjunction with the local utility company, for homeowners and utility company service providers to lower the temperature setting on the heaters. The American Academy of Pediatrics (AAP) introduced tap water scald burn prevention into their office-based anticipatory guidance program. Instead of merely exhorting parents to supervise their children more closely, the efforts targeted the adult behavioral change of walking down to the basement and turning down the temperature of the water heater. Feldman also led a campaign to pass state legislation requiring that water heaters be preset at 120–125 degrees. In 1983 the state of Washington enacted such a law.

"The focus on changing the heater (the product) rather than continued better supervision of children (changing the host) is a classic example of a passive injury prevention strategy, which works automatically once in place, in contrast to active strategies, which require repeated behavioral change on the part of individuals. The ultimate change in regulation has effectively solved the problem of these burns in young children" (Rivara 1998, 257).

The work of pediatrician Murray Katcher in Wisconsin mirrors the success of Feldman in Washington. Katcher heard Feldman present his paper on tap water scald burns at the AAP annual meeting and was struck by how a one-time action—lowering the water heater thermostat—could prevent devastating burns to children. He began his own studies, which showed that those most at risk were the physically or mentally disabled, children under 5, and adults older than 65. His initial attempts to require that manufacturers set all new hot water heaters at 120 degrees received little support, so he focused his efforts on education, working with pediatricians and other providers to educate parents on the dangers of excessively hot tap water. The local power company helped by sending education materials along with the utility bills. Most important, Katcher helped organize a strong lobbying campaign; in 1987 Wisconsin enacted a law requiring that all new water heaters be preset at 125 degrees or lower.

In other states AAP members and others formed coalitions to pass state laws. These efforts, and the threat of litigation, led to water heater manufacturers agreeing in the late 1980s to a voluntary standard that would lower the preset position.

In 1991 Ken Feldman received the AAP Practitioner Research Award for his work on tap water burns in children, and in 2003 he received the Lee Ann Miller Award from the Washington Children's Justice Conference for his impact in furthering children's justice. In 1988 Murray Katcher received the special achievements award from the AAP, and in 1997 he received a public service award from the Injury Control section of the American Public Health Association.

2.d. Andrew McGuire (1951–)

Andrew McGuire is an activist. Severely burned when he was 7 years old, as an adult in Boston in 1974 he developed the first survivor advocacy organization for burn victims and their families, which pushed for the establishment of a federal fire-resistance standard for child pajamas. Working at the Shriners Burn Institute in Boston, he sought other ways to prevent people from being burned. He became convinced that the most effective approach was to focus on cigarettes. When Andrew began the Fire-Safe Cigarette Campaign in 1979, cigarette-ignited fires caused more than one-third of all fire deaths.

In 1975 McGuire, now in California, established the Burn Council, which set up self-help groups for patients and families at six burn centers in the San Francisco Bay Area. In 1981 the Burn Council expanded its mission to include the prevention of all traumatic injuries and was renamed the Trauma Foundation.

In 1982 McGuire produced a PBS/NOVA documentary on burns entitled *Here's Looking at You Kid*. The film documented the rehabilitation of a 7-year-old boy who sustained a burn injury over 75 percent of his body; the film won an Emmy award. Another McGuire documentary told the story of a motorcyclist who was severely burned in a crash.

In the 1980s McGuire wrote proposals for the initial funding of the survivor-led organization, Mothers Against Drunk Driving (MADD), for which he also served on the first board of directors. In the late 1980s he successfully worked for the enactment of the California motorcycle helmet law. In 1982 he became a Kellogg Foundation fellow, and in 1985 he was awarded a MacArthur Foundation "genius grant."

McGuire has helped promote—sometimes successfully, sometimes not—a variety of public health initiatives in California: a seat belt law, a higher tax on cigarettes and on alcohol, improved alcohol advertising standards, and health care for battered women. In the 1990s the Trauma Foundation served as the policy center for a ten-year statewide Violence Prevention Initiative, which contributed to the passage of five gun bills in California in 1999, including a ban on the manufacture and sale of junk guns. At the turn of the century the Trauma Foundation became the coordinating agency for the Million Mom March.

McGuire's advocacy helped lead to two federal reports on fire-safe cigarettes. The first, in 1987, concluded that it was technically and economically feasible to produce a fire-safe cigarette; the second, in 1993, reported that a fire safety test method had been developed. In the late 1990s industry documents, made public as part of national tobacco litigation, revealed that it had long been possible to produce fire-safe cigarettes that consumers judged as acceptable as regular brands. The documents indicated that the industry failed to put these cigarettes into production out of concerns about liability. Beginning on June 28, 2004, New York became the first state to require all cigarettes sold there to meet the state standard for reduced ignition propensity. As of August 2008, thirty-three states (including California, Illinois, Texas, and Massachusetts) have passed similar laws.

CHAPTER 3

Work

INTRODUCTION

The vast improvement in workplace safety in the United States has been designated a twentieth-century success story by the Centers for Disease Control and Prevention (CDC 1999). Between 1933 and 1997 the unintentional work-related death rate fell 90 percent, from 37 per 100,000 to 4 per 100,000; in absolute numbers, during a century in which the workforce more than tripled from 39 million to 130 million, the annual number of workplace deaths fell from 14,500 to 5,100 (CDC 1999).

The same general forces that have led to rapid economic advances over the past two hundred years have also provided for improvements in health and safety. Many organizations have the incentive to invest in measures to reduce workplace injury and violence. It is generally good business to ensure that workers and consumers are not maimed when making or using the company product.

Many companies have health and safety programs and document their successes. The U.S. Navy, for example, writes summaries of their actions that have reduced the risk of lifting injuries, carbon monoxide poisoning, and ladder falls ("1,001 Safety Success Stories" 2007). Workers compensation specialists are paid to help industry reduce workplace problems. The Zenith Insurance Company is one of many that publicize case studies on how it helped promote safety; its work with a glass company, for example, led to a rapid reduction in worker accident claims from thirty-five per year to fourteen (The Zenith 2005).

Entrepreneurs are often rewarded for promoting safety. Every year many new products are introduced that are specifically designed to reduce accidents and injury. A recent, and unusual, innovation is a Queensland, Australia, invention to stop falling coconuts. "Getting hit on the head by a falling coconut might sound like a scene from the *Three Stooges* but in reality it is a serious problem that can have fatal results." The weight (three to four pounds) falling from sixty feet can be devastating. In the early 1980s in Papua New Guinea, being struck by a falling coconut caused 2.5 percent of trauma hospital admissions (Barss 1984). "Coconet" is a netlike device clipped to coconut trees to catch falling coconuts before they hit the ground (or the human head); it supposedly also offers economies in harvesting ("Queensland Invention" 2004).

Many occupations have their success stories. For example, during the 1980s the prevention of electrocutions became a primary emphasis of the federal government's National Institute for Occupational Safety and Health, and changes to the National Electrical Code and to Occupational Safety and Health Administration regulations, along with safety awareness campaigns by power companies and others, led to a dramatic decline in deaths due to electrocutions. During that decade work-related electrocution deaths fell from 577 per year in 1980 to 329 in 1989, from a rate of 7 per million workers to 3 per million workers—a decline of 54 percent (Stout et al 1996; CDC 1999).

A major reason for the improvement in workplace safety in the United States was a change in attitude beginning in the twentieth century, from a focus on individual worker behavior to an appreciation of the role of the employer and the work environment. For example, victim blaming was common in the early days of mine safety. During the nineteenth and early twentieth centuries operators, mine inspectors, coroners, and the courts "believed, practically as an article of faith, that miners were responsible for their own safety on the job." Concerned with explaining why miners were being killed in such large numbers, industry spokesmen and mine inspectors offered as reasons the "inevitability of accidents in a dangerous occupation, the miners' carelessness or deliberate negligence, and the lack of experience and foreign birth of many of them" (Whiteside 1990, 77). In 1886 a Colorado mine inspector stated, "I am inclined to think that disobedience, incompetence and negligence fully explain the cause of as many accidents, if not more, than are due to the hazardous character" of coal mining itself (quoted in Whiteside 1990, 79). A Utah inspector complained that "there does not appear to be any method or argument that can be advanced which will induce the miner and the workman to take proper precautions to secure their safety" (quoted in Whiteside 1990, 79). A West Virginia inspector claimed, "A personal investigation into a number of fatal accidents would almost lead to the belief that they were deliberate suicides" (quoted in Whiteside 1990, 79).

This attitude slowly changed, and over the twentieth century vast improvements were made in coal mine safety. Improved ventilation, dust suppression, safer equipment, safer work practices, and improved training all helped save workers' lives. Pick mining disappeared, and underground mining gradually gave way to surface extraction. Where miners still work underground they usually labor in highly mechanized and closely supervised operations. A major change occurred when miners won the right to organize and bargain collectively and when the piece rate system (pay per ton of coal extracted) was eliminated.

Most of the terrible mining disasters that occurred in the past two centuries resulted from methane explosions and dust fires. In the context of a highly regulated environment, managerial and engineering solutions substantially reduced the risk of these catastrophic events. Explosion-proof equipment and lights and strict smoking control policies helped remove ignition sources; improved gas and dust control through ventilation, rock dusting, and other means kept explosive mixtures from developing; and respirators and mine rescue plans and teams helped increase the odds that miners could survive explosions. Explosion-related mine fatalities declined from an average of 477 per year in 1906–1910 to under 3 per year in 1991–1995. In the twentieth century the fatal injury rate of miners from all causes fell some thirteen-fold (CDC 1999; Whiteside 1990; Stout & Linn 2002).

Explosions, fires, and other catastrophes sometimes provided the impetus for sweeping safety improvements in industry. For example, the 1911 fire in the Triangle Shirt Waist Factory, a sweatshop in Manhattan, killed 146 garment workers, mostly young immigrant Italian and Jewish women. A discarded cigarette started a fire on the eighth floor and workers on the ninth floor were trapped behind a locked exit door; the fire escape collapsed under the weight of the fleeing employees. Many workers were forced to jump from windows and ledges—to their death. The owners had a history of setting fires (when no one was at work) to "manage inventory" and thus did not install a sprinkler system that might interfere with such actions. The owners also locked many of the fire escapes to prevent theft; they estimated they were losing $25 per year. Nor were there firewalls or fireproof doors, common in New

England cotton mills. However, the owners' practices were financially rewarded; they were acquitted at trial and received large insurance payments from the fire. But the tragedy led to wide public clamor. This tragic "fire that changed America" resulted in government-mandated improvements in factory conditions, including changes to the building fire codes: requirements for multiple escape routes, outward opening doors, and sprinkler systems for higher floors (Von Drehle 2003).

The right financial incentives can spur management to improve safety practices. For example, the modern Safety First movement was born at the United States Steel Company in 1906. "U.S. Steel never ceased to claim that safety paid, both because it led to improved labor relations and because the reduction in costs far exceeded the amount spent in reducing accidents" (Aldrich, 1997, 93). Workers compensation made employers pay for workplace injuries; it is sometimes credited with transforming safety work from humanitarianism into a truly profitable activity.

Although economic incentives propelled the safety movement, the movement soon developed individuals and organizations that advanced their own safety agenda. "For safety engineers, engineering became a matter of professional standing. . . . The conclusion that injuries resulted from professional or managerial failure rather than from workers' carelessness represented a stunning reversal of earlier belief" (Alrich 1997, 121). "The shift in perspective from work accidents as routine matters of individual carelessness to the modern view that accidents reflect management failure is a measure of how much the world of work has changed in the past century. We now surround workers with a host of laws to protect their safety, and we take for granted that companies are responsible for and will take due precautions to ensure the safety of their workers" (Alrich 1997, 2–3).

Railway safety is one of the many occupations that have improved over the past century. In 1907 railroads were the nation's largest industry and a major killer; some twelve thousand people (e.g., workers, passengers, trespassers) were killed by railroads that year. By 1940 passenger risk of fatality had fallen 90 percent and worker risk by 80 percent from a half-century before. One particularly newsworthy type of accident—railroad collisions—fell some 75 percent during the 1920s, due in part to increased use of automatic block signals, which helped ensure that no other train was on that particular section of track. Other factors that led to the reduction in collisions were organizational innovation and learning, unannounced safety checks, and Safety First and other labor policies. "In addition, a host of minor modifications in equipment, signal design and operating practices continued to improve the efficiency of the block system" (Aldrich 2006, 253).

Today large companies in all industries spend substantial resources to reduce injuries among their workforce. Behavioral safety specialists emphasize the natural tendency among many people to think "It will never happen to me." And indeed, workers are correct, if "never" is replaced by "rarely." Most unsafe behavior is not immediately punished by an injury; instead, risk-taking is continually and immediately rewarded with convenience, comfort, or time saved. Because serious injuries occur rarely to any particular person, safety practices may need extrinsic support, such as intermittent praise or rewards. Safety experts stress the importance of creating a safety culture in the company, creating a sense of belonging to a community or family, where workers look out for each other (Geller 2001).

Although there have been major improvements to worker safety in the past century, much still needs to be done. The Bureau of Labor Statistics reported over 5,700 fatal occupational injuries (the leading causes of death were motor vehicle crashes and falls) and over 3 million nonfatal occupational injuries in 2006 (U.S. Department of Labor 2008). Although there are generally more job-related disease deaths than job-related injury deaths, there are more nonfatal job-related injuries than illnesses, and injuries generate more direct and indirect costs than illnesses (Leigh et al. 2000).

Every occupation has higher risks for certain injuries than for others. Some of the student papers in my Injury class have investigated the injuries occurring to such specific occupations as barbers, actors, violinists, and dentists. Hair stylists frequently cut themselves with sharp scissors; over time, their shuffling around the chair puts a burden on their lower backs and on their shoulders. One survey of Broadway performers found that 55 percent had sustained an injury in their current production; a raked stage, one that is angled down toward the audience to improve the view, is particularly hazardous for dancers (Evans et al. 1996).

Historically many injuries were designated with the name of a particular profession. For example, there was "gamekeepers' thumb," a traumatic rupture of the ligament to the thumb caused by breaking the neck of small captured prey; "hatter's shakes" caused by mercury poisoning due to the mercury and nitric acid used in the felting process; "painter's colic," caused by poisoning from lead, arsenic, mercury, turpentine, benzene, and other solvents; "flier's staleness," a syndrome that included profound apprehensions, sleep disturbances, chronic fatigue, and decreased coordination due to persistent high-altitude flying in the absence of oxygen and pressurization; and "chauffeur's knee," a partial immobility of the right knee caused by repeatedly forcing the engine crank. Other named repetitive-motion injuries are "carpetlayer's knee," "scrivener's palsy," and "telegrapher's cramp" (Cherniack 1992).

The success stories in this section include injuries to match factory workers, farmers, firefighters, construction workers, military personnel, and health care providers. They deal not only with acute injury (e.g., needlesticks) but also chronic problems caused by repetitive motion (e.g., the short-handled hoe) and continual exposure (e.g., phossy jaw). The successes involve the pre-event (e.g., train brakes), the event (e.g., tractor rollover protection), and the postevent (e.g., fires after helicopter crashes). In all the successes improving equipment or the work environment was the key to reducing injury.

The stories are presented in chronological order, in part to emphasize that progress is cumulative and that improvements in work safety have been occurring continuously over the past centuries.

WORK SUCCESS STORIES

3.1. Phossy Jaw

Phosphorus is a colorless, soft, waxy solid that glows in the dark and ignites spontaneously when in contact with air. The first friction match made from white phosphorous was produced in 1832. The first recorded cases of phosphorus necrosis ("phossy jaw") were in 1839. In 1846 a treatise was published showing that white phosphorous was poisoning workers in match factories. By the end of the century knowledge of the disease was commonplace.

Phosphorus necrosis typically led to loss of teeth, pain, swelling, and repeated dental procedures. Loss of the mandible or maxilla was common. Male patients grew beards to help hide the disfigurement. The social isolation caused by the disease was dramatic, not only because of the marked distortion of the facial features following the surgical removal of the mandible or maxilla (or both), "but because of the absolutely uncontrollable stench emanating from the sites of discharge" (Felton 1982, 98). With a 20 percent mortality rate and an induction period of only five years, phossy jaw was called "the greatest tragedy in the whole story of occupational disease" (Cherniack 1992, 371).

In 1872 Finland outlawed the use of white phosphorus matches, followed by Denmark in 1874, Switzerland in 1889, and the Netherlands in 1901. In 1906, at an international convention, France, Germany, Italy, and other European countries adopted a resolution that all parties were to prohibit the manufacture, importation, and sale of matches containing white phosphorus.

In the United States a report by the economist John Bertram Andrews in 1910, sponsored by the Bureau of Labor, reviewed findings for fifteen match plants, with clinical abstracts for many of the over one hundred patients encountered with phossy jaw. In addition to the common phosphorus poisoning of match workers, Andrews provided details on the use of phosphorus for suicide and abortions, as well as on the fatalities of fourteen child workers who died as the result of sucking or eating the match heads. (In the 1800s it was common for children to work in match factories. A child's rhyme of the nineteenth century went: "The match box, the match box/Was hard to make at three/But now I'm four or rather more/It's easier far for me.")

Andrews's report also summarized the regulatory efforts of other nations and emphasized that a harmless substitute for white phosphorus was available but that it cost a little more. Competition was so keen that a single manufacturer could not "place himself at a natural disadvantage with his rivals in business" (Felton 1982, 96).

In 1911 President Taft canceled the patent of the Diamond Match Company on nonpoisonous phosphorus sesquisulfide, and in 1912 Congress passed the Esch Act, which placed a tax of two cents per one hundred white phosphorus matches. This tax effectively eliminated the production of white phosphorus matches. The act "set a standard for workplace protection, which in many respects, has never been surpassed" (Cherniack 1992, 371).

Alice Hamilton summarized the whole long episode: "Fortunately, phosphorus poisoning in match manufacture is a thing of the past. Its abolition is an interesting story. Because the effect on the victims was so disfiguring nobody could shut his eyes to the facts. The poor creatures with distorted faces could be exhibited on the platforms at mass meetings and the whole audience won over to the cause of the abolitionists. If only lead and benzene did their work on the human face, modern industry would be much safer than it is now" (Hamilton 1925, 308–16).

LESSON: Economic incentives (e.g., taxes) can be used as a policy
measure to reduce poisoning and other injuries.

3.2. Couplers, Brakes, and Trainmen

In the early 1890s railroads were one of the major industries in the United States, and American railway workers were at high risk of injury—much higher than their European counterparts. The train crew was at particular risk; if the fatality rates of the early 1890s had continued for thirty years, about 24 of 100 trainmen would have died of injuries on the job. During this period almost half of all trainmen died performing just two tasks: coupling cars together and braking them.

Link-and-pin coupling required that the trainman stand between cars that were coming together and guide the link into the slot. Trainmen were often crushed between the mammoth vehicles. Individual hand brakes required that a trainman ride on top of the car. Many workers died when hit by overhead obstructions or when they fell from cars.

The automatic coupler, developed by Eli Janney, and the air brake, developed by George Westinghouse, were very slowly being introduced onto freight trains. In 1893 the federal Safety Appliance Act mandated the use of both these new technologies. Over the next decades learning by doing led to further improvements in the design, maintenance, and use of these devices. Between 1890–1891 and 1908–1909 the death rate per trainman from coupling fell 66 percent, and from braking (falls from cars and striking overhead obstructions) fell 53 percent.

LESSON: Technical solutions are often the most effective route to injury prevention.

3.3. Building the Golden Gate Bridge

The Golden Gate Bridge, which links San Francisco and Marin County, has been designated by the American Society of Engineers as one of the seven civil engineering wonders of the world. When it opened in 1937 it had the longest main span of any suspension bridge in existence.

The bridge was built in four years, and construction was difficult and dangerous. The Golden Gate Strait is swept by strong winds and fierce ocean currents and is often shrouded in thick fog. The bridge required the tallest towers, the longest and thickest cables, and the largest underwater foundation piers that had ever been built. The piers had to be sunk in violent open seawaters, which many thought impossible.

Yet the bridge, which cost 35 million dollars, opened ahead of schedule and under budget. At the time the norm was that a worker was killed for every million dollars spent. Given the inherent dangers and speed of the task, more than thirty-five fatalities could have been expected.

But the chief engineer, Joseph B. Strauss, insisted on the most rigorous safety precautions ever used in bridge construction. Probably the most important was the "no nonsense rule": anyone working on the bridge caught stunting, showing off, or behaving dangerously was immediately fired, a particularly severe penalty during the Great Depression. Strauss also required that protective headgear, a prototype of the modern hard hat, be worn, as well as glare-free goggles. Special face and hand cream protected workers against the wind. Men who had to climb to great heights were put on special diets to prevent dizziness.

The most conspicuous precaution was the safety net, suspended under the bridge floor from end to end. During construction the net saved the lives of nineteen workers who accidentally fell from the bridge. These men became known as the Halfway to Hell Club. By contrast, twenty-eight workers had fallen off the recently completed San Francisco Bay Bridge, and all had died.

In the first three years of construction only one man died, setting a record low for bridge fatalities. Unfortunately, on February 17, 1937, an additional ten men lost their lives when a section of the scaffold fell and broke through the safety net. Still, eleven fatalities on such a project was a safety triumph.

Ironically, through the years the Golden Gate Bridge has become the number one site in the world for suicides. Suicide experts advocate, not the replacement of the safety net, but a suicide barrier (e.g., a fence), similar to ones that have virtually eliminated suicides from the Eiffel Tower and the Empire State building. Clinical experience and much research evidence indicate that people stopped from jumping off the Golden Gate Bridge will rarely go on to kill themselves in other ways.

LESSON: It is possible to make even the most dangerous workplaces relatively safe.

3.4. Tractor Rollovers

Farmworkers are at high risk for fatal injury. Historically a significant injury problem has been tractors rolling over and crushing the driver. The risks are heightened in the case of wheeled tractors with high centers of gravity; special hazards arise when the tractor is towing other equipment. Sloping or uneven ground, soft earth, ditches, and excavations are contributing causes for rollover. Attempts to reduce the likelihood of rollover have not been very successful. For example, an engine cut-off switch to shut off power upon sensing lateral movement was introduced on tractors, but proved too slow for the dynamic forces generated in the rollover movement. However, tractors can be made so that, given a rollover, injury is less likely to occur.

The mounting of a protective frame or crush-proof cab (known as rollover protective structures, or ROPS) can prevent injuries from a tractor rollover. The desire for rollover protection started in the 1920s, as tractor rollovers became prevalent in the agricultural community. However, before 1960 few tractors had such protection. In 1959 Sweden became the first country to mandate ROPS on all new farm tractors, and despite opposition by farmers the requirement was later expanded to all existing tractors.

From the period 1957–1964 to 1986–1990 the proportion of Swedish tractors with ROPS increased steadily from 6 to 93 percent. Over that same period the tractor rollover fatality rate fell from 12 per 100,000 tractors (twenty-three fatalities per year) to 0.2 per 100,000 tractors (fewer than one fatality every two years).

LESSON: Passive (automatic) safety measures are often highly
          effective for reducing injury.

3.5. The Short-Handled Hoe

In California in the 1960s a single tool, the short-handled hoe, was responsible every year for thousands of permanent back injuries among farmworkers. The hoe, which measured eight to twenty-four inches in length, was called *el cortito* (the short one) and was used to thin weeds from delicate crops such as lettuce, strawberries, beets, celery, and carrots.

California Rural Legal Assistance (CRLA), founded in 1966, was a program in the federal War on Poverty designed to bring legal services to the disadvantaged. CRLA was staffed primarily by young activist lawyers with links to the civil rights and farmworker union movement. A lawyer with CRLA, Maurice Jourdane, recalls taking testimony on housing complaints in a California labor camp for farmworkers. One of the workers claimed, "This is bullshit: There are real problems for you to deal with, like *el cortito.*" The entire group supported his demand.

In 1972 Jourdane filed a formal complaint with the California Division of Industrial Safety (DIS), arguing that the short-handled hoe was an unsafe tool and a health hazard to farmworkers. Testimony from eleven physicians supported this claim: "When you bend over all day, the discs in your spine degenerate. In time, a disc herniates or explodes. By the time too many farm workers are forty, they're disabled or unable to work." A key piece of economic information was that the long-handled hoe was used to cultivate the same crops in every other region of the United States.

What were the growers' arguments for the short-handled hoe? At the DIS hearings the growers presented little evidence other than their own beliefs. They claimed that the short-handled hoe didn't lead to medical problems (sore and tired backs are part of hard work) and that no one had ever complained prior to CRLA intervention. In any event, workers must stoop to avoid damaging the plants. Workers saw different motives in the growers' insistence on the short-handled hoe. One worker recalled a supervisor's response to his objections to using the hoe: "With the long-handled hoe, I can't tell whether they are working or just leaning on their hoes. With the short-handled hoe I know when they are not working by how often they stand up" (quoted in Murray 1982, 28). Another worker thought that the only possible efficiency gain was because workers moved down the rows as fast as possible to get to the end so that they could rest their backs. Others thought that the growers not only tolerated injury and subsequent worker turnover, but actually preferred it. Turnover reduced the likelihood of unionization, and a steady supply of cheap Mexican labor could be relied on to fill the positions.

The DIS denied the CRLA petition on narrow grounds; they found that an unsafe or hazardous tool was one that was damaged or improperly maintained, not one that was a hazard due to its normal use: "There are, in fact, many work operations that hasten aging of various body parts at varying rates according to individual resistance" (quoted in Murray 1982, 35). But in 1975 the California Supreme Court, armed with additional information on the burden to taxpayers of unemployed Mexican American farmworkers injured by the short-handled hoe, ruled that the DIS had interpreted the regulations too narrowly.

Following the California Supreme Court ruling the demand by farmworkers that the short-handled hoe be abolished received immediate attention. Jerry Brown had replaced Ronald Reagan as governor of California in January 1975, and in April the California DIS issued an Administrative Interpretation banning the short-handled hoe.

El cortito not only caused pain and irreparable injury, but it also came to symbolize what was wrong with farmwork in California. For the workers, it was a symbol of oppression, a way to keep control of workers and make them live humbled, stooped-over lives. "For Cesar

Chavez, who played a pivotal role in the long drama, there were few greater moments than when el cortito was finally banished from California fields in 1975. In his youth, Chavez knew the hoe well, having used it to thin countless rows of lettuce. . . . Later he would say he never looked at a head of lettuce in a market without thinking of how laborers had suffered for it from seed to harvest" (Ferris & Sandoval 2006).

LESSON: Power relationships and politics affect injury rates.

3.6 Military Helicopter Fires

In many otherwise survivable aircraft accidents fire has often killed the occupants. For example, a study of almost six hundred U.S. Army helicopter accidents from 1957 to 1960 found that only 7 percent resulted in postcrash fires, but these 7 percent accounted for 63 percent of the fatalities. Ruptured fuel cells or fuel lines caused most of the fires.

The first major scientific effort to reduce the problem of *airplane* fires began in the late 1940s. The U.S. Air Force sponsored full-scale crash tests to determine if the use of low-volatility fuels offered significant safety benefits. The answer was no. The investigators also determined that no fuel tank of the era had any significant crash-resistant capabilities. During a crash fuel would often spill in liquid form from broken fuel lines and tanks and form a mist around the plane. Ignition of the mist occurred in as little as 0.6 seconds after impact, producing a fireball, usually before the plane even came to rest.

The incorporation of *helicopters* into military operations occurred during the Korean conflict (1950–1953). Little attention was paid to crashworthiness in these early years.

Crash tests of military helicopters focusing on the fuel system began in the 1960s. These tests, combined with numerous U.S. Army accident investigations, showed some of the common fuel system failures that occurred during crashes.

Following the dismal results of the wing (airplane) fuel tank tests, the Federal Aviation Administration embarked on a ten-year program to develop improved crash-resistant fuel tanks and self-sealing breakaway valves and to ensure that the fuel cells had accessories and components that would not tear the cell. In 1960 and 1961 the entire federal effort resulted in the issuance of specifications for fuel tanks and for self-sealing breakaway valves.

These standards were revised substantially over the next ten years. In 1970 the first U.S. Army helicopters with a true crash-resistant fuel system came off the production line. A study of U.S. Army helicopter accidents from 1970 to 1976 found that this system had entirely eliminated thermal fatalities and reduced thermal injuries by 75 percent in helicopter accidents. A 2002 report by the Federal Aviation Administration concluded that the military history of helicopter crash-resistant fuel systems "is outstanding. The systems work as designed, fires are prevented in survivable accidents, lives are saved and injuries reduced" (U.S. Department of Transportation 2002, 32).

Unfortunately these systems are still not in general use in civilian helicopters.

> LESSON: Engineers with a clear mission, and resources, can solve
>   even the most difficult problems.

3.7. Needlestick Injuries

Accidental needlesticks are a common and potentially serious occupational hazard for health care providers. Needlesticks can transmit HIV, hepatitis B and C, and other blood-borne diseases. An accidental needlestick can have psychological as well as physical effects on the exposed worker.

Between 1985 and 1996 the Mayo Clinic in Rochester, Minnesota, instituted numerous practice changes to reduce needlesticks for its two hundred phlebotomists. These changes included intensive safety training along with modification of the phlebotomy chairs to accommodate needle disposal on both the left and right sides of the arm post, making needle disposal buckets more accessible. Other modifications included the automatic disposal of plastic tube holders after each use, use of one-handed recapping blocks, and elimination of a double-needle technique for collecting blood culture specimens. Reducing the need to resheath used needles greatly reduced the risk of needlestick injuries.

During this period the injury rate fell from 1.5 needlesticks for every 10,000 blood draws to 0.2. In other words, because a phlebotomist can perform about 10,000 venipunctures per year, the average number of needlesticks over five years for a full-time phlebotomist fell from 7.5 to 1. Similarly, a comprehensive approach to reduce risk at Arlington Hospital in Virginia saw a 61 percent drop in needlestick injuries in a four-year period.

> LESSON: Successful injury prevention requires a comprehensive
>   approach, often with many small improvements.

3.8 Firefighter Burns

Modern plastics and other synthetic materials can cause fires to burn at higher temperatures and increase the speed of flame spread. Fortunately personal protective equipment for firefighters has improved dramatically in the past decades. Rubber jackets, rubber boots, and plastic gloves have been replaced by three-layer "bunker gear."

The New York City Fire Department is the largest fire department in the United States; in 1994 it had over eleven thousand firefighters. In 1994 the department changed to modern bunker gear, including protective overpants (traditional uniforms included only a protective overcoat). Comparing burn injury rates in 1992–1993 with those in 1995–1996, the number of lower-extremity burns decreased by 85 percent. In the month with the *lowest* number of lower-extremity burn injuries in the first two years nineteen city firefighters suffered this type of burn. In the month with the *highest* number of lower-extremity burn injuries in the two years following the introduction of modern bunker gear, ten firefighters suffered such burns. Upper-extremity burn injuries also fell markedly, by 65 percent. There were no significant changes in the incidence or severity of heat exhaustion, inhalation injuries, or cardiac events.

Evaluators concluded that "the reduction in the incidence and severity of burn injuries, the major occupational injury affecting this workforce, has been so immediate, dramatic, and without untoward effects that the introduction of the modern firefighting uniform must be characterized as a sentinel event in the history of firefighter health and safety" (Prezant et al. 1999, 479).

LESSON: Good gear can make for good health.

HEROES

3.a. Samuel Plimsoll 1824–1898

> A British Cheer for Plimsoll
> The Sailor's honest friend
> In spite of opposition
> Their rights he dares defend
> John Guest, 1875 (quoted in Jones 2006, 311)

In the mid-nineteenth century seafaring was an incredibly dangerous occupation; approximately one in five British mariners died at sea. In the decade of the 1860s alone close to six thousand ships were wrecked off the British coast. Vessels were not only often in a poor state of repair and not seaworthy, but they were commonly overloaded and unstable. Unscrupulous ship owners sometimes deliberately overloaded and overinsured these "coffin ships," risking the lives of the crew. The ship owners themselves had little risk; they garnered high profits if the ships arrived safely, and insurance money for ships that did not. Drowned sailors were easily replaced. The earl of Shaftesbury, the celebrated philanthropist, described the use of coffin ships as "one of the most terrible, the most diabolical systems that ever desolated mankind" (quoted in Jones 2006, xiv).

Samuel Plimsoll, an MP from landlocked Derby, launched a crusade to pressure Parliament, where many other MPs were ship owners, to prevent vessel overloading. He championed the simple idea of putting a line on the side of a ship to define the lowest level at which it could lie in the water. For this, his character and good name were attacked, he was sued for libel, and his health suffered. But his drive and passion made him wildly popular with the public, and he became the subject of novels, plays, and music hall songs. He also succeeded in securing the passage of the Merchant Shipping Act in 1876, which mandated maximum load lines for ships.

Plimsoll was an extraordinary man from an ordinary background. Born the son of a tax man, he worked for a decade in a brewery as a clerk and eventually the manager, then failed as a coal merchant in London and was for a time reduced to destitution. With good fortune he became an MP and eventually gave his name to the Plimsoll line, now used on ships throughout the world.

Plimsoll thrived on righteous outrage. Before he became known as "the sailor's friend" he was "the miner's friend," proposing inexpensive ways to detect gas underground and leading fund-raising efforts after mining disasters. He also campaigned in favor of public footpaths, against high railings in Regent's Park, and for the removal of fir trees that were obstructing the view of the Eden Valley.

In 1864 he survived a North Sea storm that wrecked four other ships. On investigating the norms of maritime practice, he was appalled at how many boats were overloaded and overinsured. Seamen who discovered what they had let themselves in for after signing on to a coffin ship were sent to prison for breach of contract if they refused to sail. Between 1870 and 1872 over 1,600 men were in British jails for this very offense.

Plimsoll was elected to Parliament in 1868 and for years endeavored in vain to pass a bill protecting British sailors. But his violent speeches aroused the House of Commons. In 1872 he published a book entitled *Our Seamen* that shocked the general public into clamorous indignation. His campaign was "taken up by parliamentarians, journalists, businessmen, trade unionists, novelists, playwrights, clergymen, caricaturists and music-hall performers. Its supporters flocked to meetings where they cheered its advocates and demonstrated in the streets, condemning its opponents as friends of villainy. It involved all classes of men and women alike. Florence Nightingale contributed money. Queen Victoria expressed sympathy" (Jones 2006, xi).

In the middle of his campaign an 1873 issue of *Vanity Fair* had this to say about Plimsoll:

> He is not a clever man, he is a poor speaker and a feeble writer, but he has a big good heart, and with the untutored utterings of that he has stirred even the most indifferent. He has taken up a cause, not a popular cause nor a powerful one—only the cause of the British sailor who is sent to sea in rotten vessels in order that ship-owners may thrive. He has written a book about it—a book jumbled together in the fashion of an insane farrago, written without method and without art, but powerful and eloquent beyond any work that has appeared for years because it is the simple honest cry of a simple honest man. . . . He has his reward. Any number of actions for libel have been commenced against him. . . . His crime is indeed great. He has declared that there are men among the Merchants of England who prefer their own profits to the lives of their servants, and who habitually sacrifice their men to their money.

Plimsoll lived at a time when industrial progress was largely unchecked by consumer or labor laws and when less than a tenth of the population had the right to vote. His successful campaign for maximum load lines for ships became a "milestone in the progress of people power" (Jones 2006, 61). "Samuel Plimsoll brought about one of the greatest shipping revolutions ever known by shocking the British nation into making reforms which have saved the lives of countless seamen" ("Samuel Plimsoll" 2007).

> In well known lays we sing the praise of men renown'd in war,
> How heroes brave on land and wave have fought for us of yore;
> But I will sing of one who fought, though not in deadly strife,
> The noble object that he sought was saving human life.
>
> So a cheer for Samuel Plimsoll, and let your voices blend,
> In praise of one who, truly, has proved the sailor's friend;
> Our tars upon the ocean, he struggled to defend,
> Success to Samuel Plimsoll, for he's a sailor's friend.
>
> Fred Albert, 1876 (quoted in Jones 2006, 312)

3.b. Alice Hamilton (1869–1970)

When she was young Alice Hamilton's mother said to her, "Alice, don't ever forget that there are two kinds of people in the world, the ones who say, 'Somebody ought to do something about it, but why should I?' and those who say, 'Somebody must do something about that, then why not I?'" Alice decided she was the second type of person; she was determined to make her life count (Grant 1967, 32).

Alice Hamilton chose to become a physician, in part because "as a doctor I could go anywhere I pleased, to far off lands or to city slums, and be quite sure I could be of use anywhere" (quoted in "Alice Hamilton" 2005). Her first job, teaching pathology at Northwestern University, gave her the chance to realize her dream of living at Hull House, the pioneering social settlement in Chicago, working with Jane Addams and other reformers. At the settlement house Dr. Hamilton established a well-baby clinic. She also read a book, *Dangerous Trades*, published in 1902, on hazards to the health of industrialized workers in England. She found many articles on occupational illness in Europe but nothing about such problems in the United States.

Hamilton began investigating industrial health problems. She studied the poisons affecting workers in the munitions, rubber, copper, and lead industries. She visited factories in Europe, as well as the United States, and talked with and examined workers. Her studies showed that U.S. lead factories were so dangerous that any European country would close them by law. Hamilton's studies were an essential first step in improving the working conditions in these factories, since American factory owners denied the existence of work-related diseases, let alone took responsibility for them.

Hamilton virtually always faced initial opposition: "As I look back, some striking pictures come to me of that anarchic period. One is the picture of the works manager of a big white-lead plant, a gentleman of breeding and something of a philanthropist. He is looking at me indignantly and exclaiming: 'Why, that sounds as if you think that when a man gets lead poisoning in my plant I ought to be held responsible!'" (Hamilton 1985, 4).

Hamilton pushed for a social revolution in America of the type that had already occurred in Europe: an acceptance that in the dangerous trades an employer was responsible for the health and safety of the workers.

Why did men work in the dangerous conditions that Hamilton documented?

"When we wonder why the workers did not rebel, we must remember that big industry employed almost exclusively immigrant labor at that time. In the heavy industries especially, the rule was to work the man as hard as possible—the seven-day week and twelve-hour day continued in steel until 1922—pay them as low wages as possible, and then, when American ideas began to penetrate and revolt to raise its head, to put it down with force, discharge and blacklist the trouble-makers, and start afresh with a new lot of immigrants. In this, it must be added, the heavy industries were greatly helped by the courts of law and by the state constabulary forces." (Hamilton 1985, 5) Hamilton investigated carbon monoxide poisoning in steelworkers, mercury poisoning in hatters, and "dead fingers" syndrome among laborers using jackhammers. Her combination of science, passion, and persuasion led to sweeping reforms, both voluntary and regulatory, reducing the long-term harm caused to workers. She was often able to persuade employers to do the right thing. "In her own crusade against the poisonous trades, Alice led by persuasion. She was never sarcastic, she never scolded, even when an employer was inhuman, even when a company doctor was unscrupulous" (Grant 1967, 120).

Alice Hamilton believed in progress, in reasoned discourse, and in the capacity of individuals, once informed of the facts, to take positive action. As she wrote in her autobiography, "From the first I made it a rule to try to bring before the responsible man at the top the dangers I had discovered in his plant and to persuade him to take the simple steps which even I, with no engineering knowledge, could see were needed. As I look back on it now . . . it astonishes and amuses me to see how very well this primitive method often worked. I must cite a few instances, for they redound so much to the credit of the American manufacturer" (Hamilton 1985, 8).

Her first special area of study was lead poisoning. She persuaded the National Lead Company to change its practices by convincing them that they were poisoning their own workers. She found hospital records of lead poisoning (which lacked any information about occupation), tracked down more than a score of men poisoned with lead, and showed that they were all former National Lead Company employees. The president of the company, Edward Cornish, thereupon reformed all his plants.

Most important, her science was impeccable: "In her field investigations, she applied precepts of scientific integrity and prudent public health practice that continue to influence the discipline of occupational health. These include the necessity for a strict definition of the disease problem, a thorough understanding of the industrial processes involved, and on-the-spot reporting of findings and recommendations" (CDC 1999, 462).

In 1918 Hamilton was appointed assistant professor of industrial medicine at Harvard Medical School's Department of Public Health (which was reorganized as the Harvard School of Public Health three years later). She was the first, and for many years the only woman on the Harvard faculty. As a woman, she was excluded from the Harvard Faculty Club and the commencement procession. But her work continued to promote the health and safety of American workers.

Both the National Institutes of Occupational Health and Safety and the American Public Health Association gave Alice Hamilton awards for achievements in promoting occupational health. Her picture graces a U.S. postal stamp. She was "the first American physician to devote her life to the practice of industrial medicine" (Rom 1983, 4).

3.c. John Andrews (1880–1943)

As a noted authority on occupational medicine observed, "It is only rarely that an individual is recognized for his dedication and devotion to a cause that carries no personal rewards or acclaim. . . . John B. Andrews was at the cutting edge of a movement" that targeted the prohibition of poisonous phosphorus in the manufacture of matches and other issues concerning the health and safety of workers. It is with the health of match workers "that his name is indelibly tied" (Felton 1982, 95).

In 1906 the economists Richard T. Ely and John B. Andrews founded the American Association for Labor Legislation (AALL), a research and lobbying group, which focused its resources on eradicating occupational hazards. In 1909 Dr. Andrews undertook a campaign to eliminate "phossy jaw," a painful and disfiguring necrosis of the jaw found in workers who dipped matchsticks in white phosphorus and packed them in boxes. Beginning under the auspices of the AALL, and subsequently with a contract from the Department of Labor, Andrews investigated the fifteen prime match factories around the country. Of the nearly 3,600 employees in these plants, Andrews showed that some two-thirds were subject to hazardous exposure.

After his report in 1910 Andrews led a lobbying effort to eliminate the use of white phosphorus in matches. The United States had not signed an international agreement on this toxic substance in 1906, but was now pressured into action. In 1911 the AALL induced the Diamond

Match Company, the largest U.S. match manufacturer, to assign its patent on nonpoisonous phosphorus sesquisulfide, a safe but slightly more expensive alternative, to three trustees. This act was not sufficient to allay suspicion of monopoly, however, and a few weeks later President Taft canceled the patent. Diamond Match Company then sent technicians into factories of competitors to instruct them on using the safer phosphorus.

For economists, the favorite solution to many problems is not to ban products (Europe had banned white phosphorus in matches), but to use taxes and subsidies to channel behavior. Andrews's solution in this instance was to impose a prohibitively high tax on the poisonous substance. In 1912 the U.S. government placed a heavy tax on those matches made of white phosphorus, which effectively eliminated their manufacture in this country.

During the U.S. Progressive Era (1900–1917) there was great interest in investigating and ameliorating hazardous working conditions. Andrews "orchestrated the most significant legislative success achieved by advocates of workers' health in the early twentieth century" (Young 1982, 11). His innovative tax solution resulted in "victory over phossy jaw [and] strengthened the growing belief that public concern over industrial disease could be kindled, economic roadblocks removed, and a coordinated effort by scientists and social activists achieved" ("Progressive Ideas" 2005).

3.d. Janine Jagger (1950–)

Janine Jagger, MPH, PhD, is an epidemiologist specializing in injury prevention and control. She has been devoted to reducing needlestick injuries in health care facilities, which can lead to the transmission of hepatitis B, hepatitis C, HIV, and other deadly or debilitating diseases.

Jagger's concern for medical workers caused her to shift her research from brain trauma injury to needlestick injury. "These are the people who take care of us when we are ill. And yet they are expected to put their lives and health in danger to do it. When I realized how preventable needle sticks were, I felt something had to be done" (quoted in Carlsen 1998).

In the 1980s, when Jagger began her crusade, health care workers were simply cautioned to handle sharp medical devices more carefully. With her background in automotive safety, Jagger took a public health approach. Rather than focusing on changing behavior, she advocated redesigning medical devices to reduce the potential for injury. "My idea was to try to create the equivalent of an airbag for needles" (quoted in Feigenoff 2003).

In 1988 her landmark study, published in the *New England Journal of Medicine,* showed that needlestick injuries to health care workers were more appropriately considered a device problem rather than a human problem. In her study she asked, "What stuck you?" rather than "Why did you stick yourself?" She showed that devices that required disassembly had rates of injury up to five times the rate for disposable syringes. One-third of the injuries were related to recapping. She then outlined the design criteria for safer devices that could lower the rates of injury. That pioneering research provided the foundation for the development of a new generation of safer medical devices.

Jagger did more than just study the problem. She and her colleagues currently hold five patents for safer devices. Among her various honors is the 1988 Distinguished Inventor Award from Intellectual Property Owners, Inc. The U.S. Patent and Trademark Office selected her patents for display at its 1990 Bicentennial Exhibit.

Jagger also found that no one, not the Centers for Disease Control nor the Food and Drug Administration, was collecting even the most basic statistics on the needlestick problem. No one could say, for example, how many health care workers had contracted hepatitis C or the AIDS virus from needlesticks, nor were data collected on the number of needlesticks that occurred annually in medical care facilities. So Jagger took the lead in gathering, analyzing, and disseminating information about the frequency of needlestick injuries, their circumstances, and the specific kinds of devices involved. She developed a standardized computer data system (a "surveillance system") now used by more than fifteen hundred hospitals across the country.

Jagger is the founder and first editor in chief of *Advances in Exposure Medicine,* a quarterly publication dedicated to preventing occupational transmission of blood-borne pathogens in health care. She traveled the country, appearing before committees and conferences to explain that simple needle design changes could reduce the epidemic of infections being spread through needlesticks. Jagger did more than anyone else to drive the debate over the causes and solutions to needle injuries.

On November 5, 2000, Jagger stood next to President Clinton as he signed the Needle Stick Safety and Prevention Act, requiring health care facilities to use safety-engineered needles and other sharp medical devices with protective features that retract, blunt, or otherwise shield the sharp point or edge after use.

The Advanced Medical Technology Association, the largest medical technology trade association in the world, named Jagger the "MedTech Hero" for March 2001 for her contribution to advancing medical device safety technology. In 2002 she received a MacArthur Foundation "genius grant" for her work.

Needlestick injury rates fell about 50 percent between 1993 and 2001 (Jagger & Perry 2003). Jagger cites her proudest professional moment as "seeing the needle stick rates go down and knowing that somewhere there are nurses and doctors who are leading full and healthy lives who otherwise would have been infected" (quoted in Smith 2003).

3.e. Paul O'Neill (1935–)

Paul O'Neill's emphasis on values-based leadership was based on three building blocks: (1) treat all employees with dignity and respect; (2) give them the tools, knowledge, and support they need to make a meaningful contribution to the company; and (3) recognize that contribution. When he became CEO of Alcoa in 1987 he used that philosophy to promote worker safety.

As the first outsider brought in as Alcoa CEO, O'Neill was determined to shake things up. He warned managers that they would be judged by how well they met his numbers. But O'Neill's numbers weren't the usual fare of sales growth, profit margins, or share appreciation. Instead, his sole standard was worker safety, measured by time lost to injuries. Although Alcoa already outperformed most U.S. manufacturers by this measure, O'Neill believed that if the firm wanted to become a world-class company, it first should become the safest. His declared goal was for no Alcoa employee to ever be hurt at work.

O'Neill created a culture of safety at Alcoa. At every company meeting safety was the first thing discussed. An online safety data system was created to track incidents, analyze their causes, and share information about how to prevent them from occurring again. Alcoa employees at every level were encouraged not only to report all errors, near misses, and accidents, but also to suggest solutions and improvements. Managers who did not report accidents could be terminated.

O'Neill told his managers, "Don't budget for safety. As soon as we know there is a risk, we should fix it immediately." He then gave the workers his home phone number and told them to call him if their managers did not fix safety problems. O'Neill was accessible: he worked out of a cubicle and could often be found eating lunch in the cafeteria.

To ensure that the focus on safety was a values issue, he threatened to fire any manger that brought him an analysis of how improved safety was also improving profits.

O'Neill's approach worked. Safety improved dramatically; the lost-workday rate fell over 90 percent by 2000, to less than one-twentieth of the U.S. industry average. The approach also turned out to be good for the bottom line; in 2000, when O'Neill left the firm, Alcoa had record profits of $1.5 billion on sales of $23 billion. From the time he took over the company until he left, payroll had quadrupled and profits had increased by almost six times.

O'Neill institutionalized the focus on worker safety. Alcoa's goal is now to do better than decrease the number of accidents to zero: through wellness and fitness programs, the corporation strives to send employees home healthier than they were when they came to work.

In 2001 Paul O'Neill was appointed U.S. secretary of the Treasury. During his twenty-one-month tenure there, the lost-workday rate among Treasury employees fell by more than 50 percent.

O'Neill now works with hospitals to reduce hospital infections and medication errors and improve the general quality of medical care.

CHAPTER 4

Play

INTRODUCTION

There are millions of sports and recreational injuries in the United States every year. Most are relatively minor, such as strains, sprains, scrapes, and bruises, most of which cause pain but no long-term disability. But serious injury is not uncommon. It is estimated that of the more than 20 million sports mishaps each year, over 3 million are treated in an emergency department ("A Comprehensive Study" 2003).

Four ways to reduce sports injury are to (1) improve the equipment, (2) modify the rules of the game, (3) improve the playing field, and (4) change or improve the players.

The first five stories in this section deal with improvements in equipment. The first story describes the changes in ski boots that have dramatically reduced skiing injuries. There is little need for either education about or mandating of this safety improvement, since the benefits of these boots are well known and there is little incentive not to use these superior boots.

The second success story deals with bicycle helmets that are effective in reducing head injury and death. Although it is necessary to have skis in order to ski, helmets are not a necessary part of biking, and historically, because of custom and habit, many people do not willingly wear helmets. If adult role models do not wear helmets, getting children to wear them may require more than scientific information. Mandating helmets in Victoria, Australia, has saved many children from serious head injury.

The third success story concerns bright clothing that increases visibility and reduces the risk associated with hunting. Requirements to wear hunter orange have been key to reducing accidental shootings. Such mishaps are far less common than ski falls, but potentially far more dangerous. People are not good at understanding low-probability events. Many hunters think, "No one close to me has ever been shot while hunting, so why should I change the way I dress when I hunt?" Fortunately, once a generation of hunters has become used to hunter orange, it is likely that they will feel unequipped without it.

Two success stories dealing with equipment involve face and head protection in hockey. Where they achieved maximum effectiveness, these product improvements were accompanied by rule changes mandating the equipment. Without the requirements, many players might believe they could achieve a small competitive advantage playing without the safety equipment. Rules requiring their use created a level playing field while protecting the players.

Some equipment changes that appear likely to reduce injury may do not do so. One hundred years ago John L. Sullivan, the heavyweight champion of the world, boxed bare-knuckle. The introduction of the boxing glove protected the hand but also allowed the boxers to hit harder. In Sullivan's era fights could last thirty rounds, as neither boxer punched too hard for fear of breaking his hand and losing the fight. Boxing gloves reduced that worry and permitted boxers to pummel each other, probably leading to more concussions and serious internal injuries (Hemenway 1993).

Some equipment changes that improve player performance may increase the likelihood of injury. Until the 1960s catchers' gloves were heavily padded, giving protection to the catching hand but requiring two hands to make a catch. Then in the 1960s catchers began using thinner gloves so that they could catch with one hand, making it easier for them to get to the ball quickly to throw out a stealing base runner. Unfortunately the repetitive trauma from continually catching pitched balls with thinner gloves leads to damage of the gloved hand (e.g., diminished blood flow, swelling of the index finger).

Changing the rules of the game is often an effective way to reduce injuries. Two football success stories illustrate the importance of making rules that protect rather than endanger players. One of these changes was necessitated by a supposed improvement in helmets, which led coaches to change the way they taught players to tackle. The other change occurred a century ago and dramatically altered the way football was played.

My grandfather, Clarence "Skinny" Wilson, was a fine athlete; he was born in 1888 and played semi-pro baseball and football. I remember him telling me how, as a teenager, when his football team got close to the goal line, they would give him the ball and then literally throw him over the goal line for a touchdown. An NCAA rule change in 1905 made that maneuver illegal.

It is possible to reduce injury by altering the playing field. In football, for example, wooden goal posts used to be placed on the goal line; they were unpadded and easy to run into during the game. Padding was eventually placed on the posts, and then, wisely, the two posts were merged into a single post and the structure was placed outside the end zone, where it is unlikely that anyone will crash into it. In football certain types of artificial surface lead to more injuries than grass. A study in the 1980s by some of my students found that there were 30 percent more National Football League players on the injured reserve list the week after a game on "tartan turf" compared to when they played on grass (Solnick & Calvert 1989). Reverting to grass surfaces or making the artificial surfaces softer can reduce injury. Similarly, for softball, studies show that changing from the popular "Hollywood bases" to breakaway bases would dramatically reduce injuries to the hands and feet (Janda et al. 1990).

In terms of the players themselves, a number of changes can be implemented, including selection (e.g., don't let small children play hardball), education (e.g., improving cognitive ability), and, perhaps most important, training (e.g., getting in shape). Education or training is sometimes the first (and only) policy considered to reduce injury, but other policies are often more cost-effective, especially for activities involving children. If education was all it took to change behavior, a game such as Mother May I?, which tests whether a child can remember to say three simple words, would not exist.

Evidence shows that the well-intentioned Eddie Eagle GunSafe program, which was created to educate children about the dangers of firearms, does little either to change their behavior or to improve their safety. Eddie Eagle teaches children to follow four rules if they see a gun: stop, don't touch, leave the area, and tell an adult. Although some children are able to verbalize this message, controlled studies find that they are no less likely than children who did not receive the training to handle a gun or to pull the trigger (Hemenway 2006).

Other success stories in this section deal with recreational activities. Children in the inner city sometimes play barefooted (and barehanded) and can easily cut themselves on broken glass. Any policy that reduces the glass in their playing areas (e.g., the Massachusetts bottle bill) can reduce injury. The improvements in playgrounds in Harlem led to a dramatic reduction in unintentional injuries to children, as did improvements to playgrounds in Toronto. Banning a very dangerous product, such as lawn darts, can also reduce childhood injuries.

Enforcing reasonable rules of behavior can reduce injuries. Community mobilization, including increased local enforcement, has had success in decreasing high-risk automobile driving and alcohol-related motor vehicle injuries (Holder et al. 2000). The final success story in this section describes a communitywide effort to reduce illegal and high-risk behavior by snowmobile drivers. Enforcement of rules and regulations can improve safety, but enforcement is rarely the only way to reduce injuries, and it is not always the most cost-effective policy.

PLAY SUCCESS STORIES

4.1. Ski Boots and Bindings

In the 1960s most ski injuries were to the lower extremities. These injuries tended to be more serious than those to the upper body; sprained ankles and fractured tibias were common. Progressive improvements in the ski boot, such as providing increased support for the ankle, and a decline in the average release torque of the bindings, which also reduced twist-related problems, dramatically reduced lower leg injuries from skiing. After improvements were made in the boots and bindings, injuries per 1,000 skier days at Mt. Snow, Vermont, fell from 5.9 in the 1960–1961 season to 3.4 in 1972–1973. At Sun Valley, Idaho, injuries per 1,000 skier days fell from 7.4 in 1960–1961 to 3.2 in 1972–1973 to 2.6 in 1975–1976. The reductions were primarily due to reduced rates of lower leg injuries. Ski equipment improvements continued throughout the 1970s. At Sugarbush North, Vermont, from 1972–1973 to 1980–1981 ankle sprain injuries fell 82 percent, and tibia fractures 69 percent; there was no change in upper body injuries, as no development in the sport was designed to reduce injuries there. Ski areas in other countries also reported dramatic reductions in lower leg injuries between the 1960s and the 1980s.

In the 1960s ambulances used to line up at ski areas to shuttle the injured skiers to local medical facilities. By the 1980s, these lines of ambulances were a thing of the past, a relic of a more dangerous era.

LESSON: Technological safety improvements often occur without
(the threat of) governmental intervention.

4.2. Bicycle Helmets

Bicycle helmets can substantially reduce serious injury and death. A meta-analysis of thirteen peer-reviewed studies found that wearing helmets reduced the likelihood of head injury by 60 percent. Head injury is the cause of death in the large majority of bicycle fatalities.

On July 1, 1990, the state of Victoria, Australia (which includes Melbourne), with a population of 4.3 million, instituted a law requiring that all bicyclists wear an approved safety helmet. The law was preceded by a decade-long campaign to promote the importance of helmet use. Average rates for helmet-wearing in Victoria rose from 5 percent in 1982–1983 to 31 percent in 1989–1990, jumped to 75 percent in 1990–1991 following the introduction of the law, and continued to rise, to 83 percent by the middle of 1992.

In 1982–1983 there were over 120 severe bicycle head injuries in Victoria. That number had fallen by over 50 percent by 1989–1990. Between 1989–1990, the twelve months before the law was enacted, and 1991–1992 the number of bicyclists with head injuries in Victoria fell an additional 70 percent. Overall cycling rates stayed about the same: bicycling decreased for children following the law, but increased for adults.

> LESSON: What's in the head is what separates humans from other animals, and humans are the only animals that can really protect their heads.

4.3. Hunter Orange

A danger in hunting is being shot when mistaken for game. "Hunter orange" is a florescent or blaze orange that has been shown to increase one's visibility to other hunters. It is a color not seen in nature.

Beginning in 1987 North Carolina hunters were required to wear hunter orange clothing while in the woods. Comparing the four years before the law with the four years after, gunshot deaths of hunters "mistaken for game" fell from twelve to two, while hunters accidentally shot and killed for other reasons remained constant at twenty-two. In New York between 1989 and 1995 508 hunting-associated injuries were reported; of these, 125 occurred when the injured hunter was mistaken for game. Although the vast majority of New York hunters were wearing hunter orange, 94 percent of those mistaken for game were not. Most states now require, and all strongly encourage, hunters to wear hunter orange. Fortunately, what is so bright to human eyes is not similarly bright to most game animals; deer seem to have difficulty distinguishing orange from green.

LESSON: Clothes can save the man.

4.4. Hockey Eye Injuries

In the 1972–1973 season, when data were first compiled, hockey players in Canada suffered 287 eye injuries, including 20 injuries severe enough to cause blindness. In the late 1970s regulations required that in minor hockey, all players (amateurs ages 3–20) had to wear full-face protection. Currently in major junior (youth professional) hockey half-visors are compulsory; no eye protection is required in the National Hockey League or in adult hockey. Between 1972 and 2002, 311 blindings were recorded among hockey players in Canada, only 8 of these to players wearing certified half-visors and none to players wearing a certified full-face protector.

Because of better facial protection, rule changes (e.g., no high sticking), changes in coaching techniques, and larger ice areas, reported eye injuries in Canadian hockey fell from 287 in 1972–1973 to 6 in 2000–2001, and the number of blindings fell from 20 to 1.

LESSON: Sports should be fun without being overly dangerous.

4.5. Goalie Masks

Jacques Plante (Jake the Snake) was one of the most important goalies in National Hockey League history: he changed the way goalies played—and looked. Indeed, it can be said that he changed the face of hockey. From 1955 to 1960 Plante was the goalie for the Montreal Canadiens dynasty, which won five Stanley Cup championships in a row. In each of those years Plante also won the Vezina Trophy, the top award for goalies, as he allowed the fewest goals per game. Plante's roaming style of play was innovative; he often moved out of the crease, for example, to handle the puck behind the net for his defensemen on shoot-ins.

On November 1, 1959, at the old Madison Square Garden, Plante was struck in the face by a shot from the New York Rangers' Andy Bathgate. The game was delayed while Plante, his face bleeding and swollen, received seven stitches. The goalie told his coach he would not return to the game without a mask, one he had sometimes worn in practice. The coach opposed the idea, but without a backup goalie, he relented. A masked Plante returned to the ice, shocking a sell-out crowd and the Ranger players. In the following years Plante continued to wear the mask; he was ridiculed, called a coward, and had to endure taunts about his manhood.

Plante was the first NHL goalie to wear a mask in almost thirty years, and the first NHL goalie to wear one for more than two games. The Canadiens were on a seven-game unbeaten streak when Plante donned the mask; that streak continued to eighteen, as a masked Plante went 10–0-1 in November. The Canadiens went on to win their fifth straight Stanley Cup, and Plante the award for the best goalie. Plante won the Vezina Trophy again in 1962 and 1969. In 1962 he was awarded the Hart Memorial Trophy as the most valuable player in the entire league.

By the mid-1960s headgear was widespread among NHL goalies. The last NHL goalie to play without a mask did so in 1973.

LESSON: Change is hard; it's easier when change is led by the best.

4.6. Cervical Quadriplegia from Football Injuries

Improvements in football helmets and facemasks in the 1960s and early 1970s reduced the danger of broken noses, lost teeth, and ocular damage. Unfortunately the stronger helmets led to changes in blocking and tackling. Players were taught to use their head as the primary point of contact, leading to an increase in cervical injury with quadriplegia. Most of the high school and college players who were rendered quadriplegic sustained their injuries while attempting to make a tackle. Defensive backs and specialty team players were at particular risk. As a result, college and high school athletic associations changed the rules in 1976, penalizing teams when players used their helmets to spear or butt. Coaching techniques quickly changed to eliminate the use of the head as a battering ram. The result was a dramatic reduction in the incidence of quadriplegia in high school and college football, from twenty-eight cases in 1975 to five cases in 1984.

LESSON: The rules of the game can be changed to reduce injury.

4.7. Harvard Football

Early American football was a tough sport; all plays were running plays (there was no forward pass) and players wore few pads. Many injuries occurred in the "bunch" or "pile," which formed after a player running with the ball was tackled. After the 1905 season the National Collegiate

Athletic Association made sweeping rule changes designed to open up the game, reduce the number of "mass plays," and lower the injury rate. These changes included approving the forward pass and increasing the number of yards required for a first down from five to ten. In addition, various maneuvers were eliminated, including hurdling, tripping, striking a player in the face with the heel of the hand, and striking with locked hands. A third official was added to watch for infractions.

Team physicians at Harvard University had carefully documented the injury problem among players on the varsity squad in the 1905 season; one of their conclusions was that "the percentage of injury is much too great for any mere sport." These data helped spur the NCAA rule changes, as did the fear of government action if the high injury rates continued. Three years later the Harvard doctors compared the serious injuries to Harvard varsity players in 1905 (before the changes) with those in 1906–1908 (after the changes). Fractures fell from 29 to 5 per year, dislocations from 28 to 3, ankle sprains from 13 to 4, concussions (all involving a loss of memory) from 19 to 4, and overall injuries from 145 to 38. The physicians credited not only the rule changes, but better training and increased use of protective gear for reducing the number and severity of the injuries.

LESSON: Data are crucial both in highlighting the problem and in evaluating the effectiveness of interventions.

4.8. Broken Glass Lacerations

For many years in the United States lacerations were the most common pediatric injury that required evaluation by a physician. Broken bottle glass was generally the leading cause of these lacerations; for example, broken glass bottles accounted for 15 percent of lacerations seen in an emergency department at an urban children's hospital.

In January 1983, in an effort to reduce litter and increase conservational recycling, Massachusetts enacted legislation requiring mandatory monetary deposits on beverage containers. Instead of being left on the sidewalk, bottles were brought back for the deposit. The law reduced the amount of glass bottles in the environment and injuries due to broken glass. Between 1980 and 1982, Children's Hospital in Boston treated a steady yearly average of about 110 children for glass-related lacerations occurring outside the home. In 1983 that number fell to 38. The number of children treated for fractures, for non-glass-related lacerations, and for glass-related lacerations occurring at home either stayed the same or increased slightly. There were no organized outdoor Boston clean-up programs during this period. The conservational "bottle bill" legislation had the beneficial side effect of reducing urban children's exposure to and injuries from broken glass.

LESSON: Laws enacted for other purposes can have effects on the
              likelihood of injury.

4.9. *Child Injuries in Harlem*

In 1988, Harlem Hospital in New York City admitted 273 children (ages 5–17) with severe injuries. Many were being injured by broken, rusty equipment on school and park playgrounds. Others were struck by cars while playing in the streets after school; there were few organized sports or afterschool programs for them.

In 1988 the Harlem Hospital Injury Prevention Program began documenting the unsafe conditions in Harlem parks, playgrounds, and schoolyards: the dangerous equipment, unpadded surfaces, rodent infestation, and drug dealing. The program worked with community groups, schools, foundations, city agencies, and neighbors and parents to upgrade play areas and build new ones. In 1991 not a single child was admitted to Harlem Hospital for a swing injury, which had previously been the major cause of equipment-related park and playground injuries.

Intensive educational programs were established for violence prevention and traffic safety. Smoke detectors and bicycle helmets were distributed either free or at reasonable cost in the community. An array of afterschool sports and arts programs were organized and expanded, including a hospital-based art studio and dance clinic, Little League teams, a soccer league, and a winter baseball clinic. By 1996 the annual number of child injury admissions at Harlem Hospital had fallen from 273 to 120. The declines were largest for the specific problems on which the program focused.

LESSON: Sometimes the crucial step is to recognize that something
              can be done.

4.10. *Playground Injuries*

In 1998 the Canadian Standards Association (CSA) revised their standards for safe playgrounds. Using these standards, the Toronto District School Board worked with a playground consultant to assess all playground equipment in its almost four hundred elementary schools for CSA compliance. The assessment identified many schools with playground equipment that represented an immediate risk of serious injury (e.g., the risk of falling from a height unto concrete). In close to one hundred of these schools the equipment was removed in the summer of 2000 and replaced within a year and a half with equipment meeting the standards.

Before replacement, students (ages 4–11) in these schools with hazardous equipment had rates of playground injuries serious enough to require medical attention that were 80 percent higher than in other schools. With the new, safer equipment, the injury rates in these schools fell and became equivalent to the other schools. In the first year this meant a reduction of more than five hundred playground injuries (Howard et al. 2005). Impact-absorbing surfaces and other playground improvements have also helped reduce injuries to children in many other countries.

LESSON: Kids can play, explore, have fun, and still be safe.

4.11. Lawn Darts

Lawn darts, also known as yard darts or Jarts, is an outdoor game similar to horseshoes. The darts measure about a foot long, with a long metal tip and plastic fins. Although the tip is blunt, the darts strike the ground with an estimated force of 23,000 pounds per square inch. Structurally, lawn darts are comparable to fléchettes, small steel aerial darts used as weapons in World War I.

In the 1980s 500,000 to a million lawn dart sets were sold each year in the United States and were responsible for over 650 emergency department visits per year. Three-quarters of all injuries were to children. A majority of the injuries were to the head, eye, or face; over 20 percent of all emergency department visits involved a dart penetrating the skull; and the worst injuries resulted in unilateral blindness or brain damage. Three children were killed between 1970 and 1987.

In 1970 the Food and Drug Administration ruled that lawn darts were to be sold as an adult game with warning labels and could be sold only with sporting goods, not with toys. But compliance seems to have been incomplete, with the warnings barely visible.

In 1987 a 7-year-old girl was killed in Riverside, California, by a lawn dart. She was playing alone in the front yard with her dolls when she was struck in the head by a stray dart thrown from a neighboring property. The dart set had come as a free accompaniment to a volleyball set. The girl's father, David Snow, quit his job as an aeronautics production supervisor at Hughes Aircraft and spent the next eighteen months in a tireless campaign to prevent additional children from being injured by lawn darts.

A year and a half later, within a week of each other, the Consumer Product Safety Commission and Congress both passed a ban on the sale of lawn darts. The ban was so quickly passed because there was little opposition: total retail sales in the United States at that time were only $5 million to $7 million, and there was only one U.S. manufacturer. Lawn darts was a game of limited recreational value, and safer alternatives, such as plastic horseshoes and beanbag games, easily met consumers' needs.

LESSON: "There is no power like that of parents assuaging grief"
(Will 1988).

4.12. Snowmobiling

Snowmobiling is a popular winter sport, enjoyed by more than 2 million North Americans. The modern snowmobile can weigh in excess of six hundred pounds and travel at speeds exceeding ninety miles per hour. In the first decade of the twenty-first century snowmobile accidents led to approximately two hundred deaths of Americans and Canadians each year and fourteen thousand injuries. A Canadian study found that among winter sports and recreational activities in 2000–2001 snowmobiling was the leading cause of severe injury and death in Canada, surpassing downhill skiing and snowboarding combined. Alcohol, speed, darkness, and off-trail riding are among the common factors in snowmobile deaths.

Prior to the 1993–1994 season, Sudbury, a northern Ontario community with high rates of snowmobile trauma, created the Snowmobile Trial Officer Patrol (STOP). The STOP program carefully selected and trained volunteer deputized provincial officers to patrol local trails, promoting safety, enforcing regulations, and assisting police with sobriety spot checks and alcohol interdiction efforts. In each of the subsequent three years the eleven STOP constables checked over two thousand vehicles and issued approximately four hundred warnings.

In the three pre-STOP years there were a total of fifteen snowmobile deaths in this community of about 160,000. In the three post-STOP years the number of deaths fell to four. Nonfatal snowmobile injuries serious enough to require admission to the hospital fell from eighty-seven to fifty-three. Weather conditions during these two periods were similar. Other regions in Canada did not experience this type of decrease in snowmobile injury.

LESSON: Increased enforcement can help reduce inappropriate
              behavior and resulting injury.

HEROES

4.a. Tom Pashby (1915–2005)

After finishing medical school, in 1941 Tom Pashby entered the Royal Canadian Air Force. He conducted eye tests on would-be pilots and bombardiers and became interested in ophthalmology. After the war, in 1948, he opened his own practice.

At a Saturday morning hockey game in 1959 his eldest son, age 13, was carrying the puck when he was checked from behind. The boy fell, striking his bare head on the ice. He swallowed his tongue but was saved from suffocation by the quick action of a doctor in the stands. The boy also suffered a severe concussion and a broken collarbone. He was raced to the hospital, where his father happened to be on duty.

That terrible morning, during which his son was unconscious, so disturbed Pashby as to change his life. "The close call led to a life-long search for a means to halt such potentially catastrophic injuries. Dr. Pashby's quest became a campaign and, eventually, a crusade" (Hawthorn 2005).

Tom Pashby decided he would not let his sons play hockey without a helmet. He was doing work with the Toronto Maple Leafs at the time, and Bert Olmstead, a left winger, helped him get a decent helmet from Sweden. Pashby's youngest son is believed to be the first player in the Toronto Hockey League to wear a helmet; his father told him, "You wear that helmet or you don't play." That primitive headgear is now part of the Hockey Hall of Fame.

Pashby faced a battle to change the culture of a sport that regarded the wearing of a helmet as the sign of a sissy. However, by 1965 he had helped induce the Canadian Amateur Hockey Association to make the wearing of helmets mandatory in minor hockey.

The original helmets, however, were not ideal from either a safety or an aesthetic perspective. In 1975 Pashby became chair of the Canadian Standards Association committee that approved hockey equipment. Canadian standards for hockey helmets were developed for the first time, and in 1976 the Canadian Amateur Hockey Association mandated that all amateur players wear CSA-certified helmets. In 1979 the National Hockey League made helmets mandatory for all rookie players.

Early on, when Pashby looked for statistics on serious hockey injuries he found few, so he began collecting them himself. He was astonished at the number of career-ending injuries he was able to document. In the early 1970s, on his own initiative, he surveyed all of Canada's ophthalmologists and found that in a single season there had been over 250 hockey eye injuries, with more than 40 blindings. The average age of the victims was 14.

Pashby pioneered the development of visors and wire facemasks in hockey. In 1979 his CSA committee created standards for facial protectors, and in 1980 the Canadian Amateur Hockey Association required that all minor players wear the certified protectors. In the past twenty-five years no player has ever been blinded wearing an approved full-face protector.

Pashby also lobbied successfully to make checks from behind and checks to the head illegal. The Canadian Amateur Hockey Association (now Hockey Canada) made both changes.

"Over the years, he overcame hockey's macho posturing, as helmets and visors became as much a part of a player's equipment as skates and a stick. Generations of hockey players, from professionals in the National Hockey League to weekend warriors playing pickup, owe their health, their eyesight and, in some cases, their lives to his unwavering advocacy" (Hawthorn 2005). Dr. Pashby received the Order of Canada in 1981 and an honorary doctorate from the University of Waterloo. In 2000 he was inducted into Canada's Sports Hall of Fame.

"Dr. Pashby's contribution to the betterment of society is immeasurable. He was a pioneer in the development of standards for sports and his impact on CSA and Canadian standards development will be felt for generations. For many years his portrait has hung in the entrance to CSA Group headquarters as a reminder of the impact one person can make toward the safety of all Canadians" ("Standards Pioneer" 2005).

4.b. Paul Vinger (1939–)

Paul Vinger is an ophthalmologist working in private practice in Lexington, Massachusetts. Through the years he has devoted at least a quarter of his time to pro bono public health work, helping to reduce eye injuries.

Eye injuries—at work, in the military, during sports—are a serious problem in the United States. Many years ago Dr. Vinger created a laboratory in his basement to help study the effects on human eyes of various projectiles (e.g., tennis balls, hockey pucks). He also worked tirelessly to help write consensus standards for protective eyewear, help certify safe equipment, and promote safe rules for sports.

Safety in sports doesn't just happen. The equipment has to be safe and the rules have to promote safety. In the early 1970s many sports lacked good safety standards for their equipment. Such standards are often written by nonprofit organizations such as the American Society for Testing and Materials. In 1973 Vinger was the founding member of the Eye Safety Subcommittee of ASTM, for which he continues to volunteer his expertise.

A problem for sports injury prevention is that even after standards are written and a credible certification agency is created, tradition-bound resistance may prevent beneficial change. Vinger has worked with many schools and associations of schools, prodding them to institute rule changes that prevent eye injuries. Even so, experts believe that almost all sports-related eye injuries are readily preventable.

Vinger's goal has always been to help prevent injuries while maintaining the enjoyment of the sport. For example, in the early 1980s people mistakenly thought that ski or shop goggles would provide sufficient protection against paintball injuries. That was incorrect. Under liability pressure from eye-injured participants, the paintball industry went to the ASTM for help. The ASTM formed a task force in 1994 and wrote safety standards for equipment and rules. Today "it's safer to play paintball with protection on an accredited field than it is to play badminton in your backyard," says Vinger, who cofounded the Protective Eyewear Certification Council that certifies whether eye protection for many sports, including paintball, meets the ASTM standard. However, Vinger believes that certain equipment should be banned. He has worked within ASTM to eliminate the use of fully automatic markers, which can fire fifteen to twenty paintballs per second (McConnell 2004).

An article on Harvard's Massachusetts Eye Research and Surgery Institute website reports that approximately 100,000 sports-related eye injuries occurred in the United States in 1996; it is estimated that 90 percent could have been prevented by appropriate eye protection. Without the work of Vinger and others like him, the number of injuries would have been much higher. "One of the pioneers in this area, Dr. Paul Vinger, of Lexington Eye Associates in Lexington, Massachusetts, was almost single-handedly responsible for legislation requiring protective face and eye wear in school hockey programs" (Foster 1996).

An editorial in the *British Journal of Ophthalmology* on the reduction of soccer (football) ocular injuries emphasizes the importance of the sports eyewear standards, written largely by the ASTM. The editorial concludes, "In the final comment of this editorial we have to honor Dr. Paul Vinger for all the work developed in sports ophthalmology. Dr. Vinger has devoted years of research time to the study of eye injuries, their mechanism and prevention. These studies have led to the establishment of standards of eye protective equipment in racket sports, ski goggles, hockey face helmets, baseball face protectors, fencing headgear, equestrian head protection, paintball, and since this issue of BJO, soccer eye protection" (Capao Filipe 2004, 160).

There is nothing that assures that sports will be as beneficial to youth as they could be. Data on sports injuries are not always collected. There are not enough people doing research on ball velocities or eye strength. Some protective equipment is inadequate. Some coaches are poorly trained in injury prevention. Fortunately, there are people like Paul Vinger who are willing to sacrifice time and income to try to make the world a better and safer place. In 1996 Dr. Vinger was presented the Award of Merit by ASTM, and in 1998 was the guest of honor at the annual meeting of the American Academy of Ophthalmology.

4.c. Barbara Barlow (1938–)

Barbara Barlow grew up in bucolic Pennsylvania Amish country. She changed her plans to become a medical missionary abroad when she did a surgical residency in the Bronx and decided she wanted to provide poor children in the United States with the same quality of medical care that middle-class children received. She became the first full-time pediatric surgeon at Harlem Hospital Center.

In the 1970s Barlow was treating a dozen children each year who had fallen from windows. Convinced that prevention was better than waiting for such terrible tragedies to happen, she put her energy into the city health department's "Children Can't Fly" window guard campaign. Children were sent home from the hospital clinics with window-guard request forms. Parents installed the guards and injuries and deaths from window falls decreased dramatically. At the culmination of the campaign "Children Can't Fly" balloons were tied to window gates all over Harlem.

If window falls could be prevented, thought Barlow, so could other kinds of traumatic injuries. She next turned her attention to Harlem's dirty and dangerous playgrounds.

It was apparent that Harlem children had no safe place to play outside. The concrete playgrounds were filled with broken glass, drug dealers, and

weapons. So the children played in the streets, where they were sometimes hit by cars or caught in gunfights. Children were being injured at
an alarming rate. Barlow decided that the children needed good playgrounds with adult supervision and that the hospital and the community could do something about it. At the time this was a radical concept.

Traditionally, hospitals wait for problems to come to them; instead,
Barlow went out into the community to prevent the problems from occurring in the first place. She helped put together a hospital-community coalition, which assembled injury data and took photos of the rusty equipment
and unsafe conditions of the playgrounds. With the Harlem Hospital and
Columbia University behind them, the coalition took their evidence to the
city and to potential donors (e.g., foundations, corporations).

One by one, dozens of playgrounds were rebuilt and repaired. For
example, after six years of fund-raising, the Harriet Tubman School playground got its makeover. The city provided half the funds, and Coca-Cola
Corp. the other half. But it was the neighbors who actually built the playground, turning out for a weekend construction party hosted by a local
social service organization, the school parents association, and Coca-
Cola. Earlier, the parents had met with the playground designer to tell her
exactly what the community needed.

Barlow's coalition would not rebuild a playground unless there was
strong community participation. If the community builds it, then they
feel they own it. Barlow cites the most incredible day of her life as a
Saturday she and seventy-five parents from the community built a playground in a neighborhood public school. She likened it to a Pennsylvania
barn-raising; some parents took care of the food, some the tools, and all
worked together.

Barlow's coalition used the same strategy to organize and expand a
wide array of safe and creative activities for children and youth, including weekend dance and arts clinics at the hospital, a bike club, and Little
League teams. Initially funded by grants from the Robert Wood Johnson
Foundation and Harlem Hospital, the coalition lobbied individuals,
corporations, and foundations for each specific project.

Success breeds success. As the project started getting publicity, newspapers and magazines wrote lovely articles and people sent checks.
Between 1988 and 1998 such activities helped sharply reduce children's
injuries in Harlem. In a decade the community's playground injury rate
went from twice the national average to half the national average. Said
Barlow in the late 1990s, "If someone told me that we could prevent
child injuries and find the money to rebuild all the playgrounds in central

Harlem, I would have never believed them. You never know what you can do until you try" (quoted in Howerton 1998, 2).

Barlow believes that the greatest barrier to child safety is "the idea that injuries are accidents and not a health problem. Often we deal with parents and families who think that injuries are an act of God, rather than a result of circumstance and a poor recreational environment. The reality is: injuries are preventable. Our research shows this" (quoted in "Q & A" 2002, 1–2).

In 2001 Barlow received the Distinguished Career Award from the American Public Health Association and in 2003 the Distinguished Women in Medicine Award from the National Institutes of Health.

CHAPTER 5

Nature

INTRODUCTION

Natural disasters include avalanches, blizzards, earthquakes, floods, hail, heat waves, hurricanes, landslides, thunderstorms, tornadoes, tsunamis, volcanoes, wildfires, and windstorms.

Natural disasters have played an important role in world history. In 1274, for example, Kublai Khan, ruler of the Mongol empire, was preparing to invade the island of Japan. Fortunately for the Japanese, a powerful storm sunk three hundred of his one thousand ships, killing about one-third of his forty thousand troops. Not to be deterred, in 1281 Khan set forth with a much larger force of 150,000 men to invade Japan. Another storm struck his great fleet, sinking four thousand vessels, taking 100,000 lives, and sparing Japan. Not surprisingly, Japan considered the two great storms as signs of divine protection. Seven hundred years later, near the end of World War II, when they faced the next truly serious threat of invasion, the Japanese organized suicide squadrons of kamikaze, after the name given these two fateful storms: "divine wind" (Sheets & Williams 2001).

Natural disasters have killed many millions throughout history, from the destruction of Pompeii, the Roman city buried during a catastrophic eruption of the volcano Mount Vesuvius in AD 79, to the Mediterranean earthquake in 1201 that killed more than one million people in Egypt and Syria. In more recent times, a 1970 tropical cyclone killed some 300,000 people in what is now Bangladesh; a 1976 earthquake in

TABLE 2
Deaths from natural disasters, United States

	Deaths from Lightning (per year)	Deaths from Tornadoes (per year)
1940s	329	179
1950s	184	141
1960s	133	94
1970s	98	99
1980s	73	52
1990s	57	58
2000–2004	44	45

SOURCE: National Weather Service website, http://www.nws.noaa.gov/om/hazstats.shtml. Accessed July 2005.

Tianjin, China, killed more than 250,000 people; and in December 2004 an Indian Ocean earthquake lead to a tsunami that is estimated to have killed over 240,000 people.

In the United States, by contrast, the National Weather Service reported 369 weather-related fatalities in 2004. The big killers were flooding, tornadoes, hurricanes, rip currents, and lightning. Extreme heat, which has been the major U.S. weather-related killer in recent decades, claimed only six lives (National Weather Service 2005).

The number of deaths due to natural disaster has been falling for decades in the United States. Lightning fatalities, for example, fell from over three hundred per year in the 1940s to fewer than fifty per year in the first decade of the twenty-first century (Table 2). There were almost as many deaths per year from lightning strikes in the 1940s as there currently are from all natural disasters combined.

Unfortunately huge disasters can still occur. In September 2005 Hurricane Katrina devastated parts of Mississippi, Louisiana, and other Gulf Coast states, virtually destroying New Orleans. Inadequate protection and evacuation, along with slow relief efforts, led to many more deaths than should have occurred. Still, over the past century, we have generally been getting better in dealing with natural disasters.

The stories in this section show how we have increased our ability to deal with hurricanes, icebergs, volcanic eruptions, tsunamis, and snow avalanches. We have not been able to control many forces of nature, though we can limit some, such as floods and mudslides. But we have substantially increased our ability to predict potential disasters. The first four stories show the importance of knowing when and where natural catastrophes may occur, and then what to do. These stories deal with keeping people out of harm's way. The final success story deals with the postevent, rescuing people who have been caught in dangerous snow avalanches. Avalanche transceivers (beacons) make it easier to quickly locate possible survivors.

NATURE SUCCESS STORIES

5.1. Iceberg Patrols

The Grand Banks in the North Atlantic is a hazardous and dynamic environment characterized by poor visibility (70 percent cloud or fog). For about six months a year icebergs are a grave threat to vessels. For example, between 1882 and 1890 fourteen ships were lost and forty seriously damaged in the vicinity of the Grand Banks due to collisions with icebergs. Including whaling and fishing vessels would markedly increase that total. It took one of the greatest marine disasters of all time—the sinking of the *Titanic* on April 15, 1912—to incite the public to demand international cooperation to deal with this marine hazard.

The *Titanic,* the largest movable human-made object of its era, had the latest safety features, such as automatically closing watertight doors. The press called her unsinkable. Yet on her maiden voyage she struck an iceberg in clear skies and calm seas and sunk completely within 2.5 hours, killing about fifteen hundred of her complement of over two thousand crew and passengers.

Thirteen nations involved with shipping in the treacherous North Atlantic came together to prevent further catastrophes. Their approach was simple but effective: they would all pay to ensure that the portion of the transatlantic shipping lanes threatened by icebergs would be guarded by observers who would report the location and movement of all ice. (Through the years, destruction of dangerous icebergs has been attempted but with little success.)

From its inception until the beginning of World War II, the International Ice Patrol was conducted from two surface patrol cutters. Since World War II aerial surveillance has become the primary ice reconnaissance method. Up to one thousand icebergs are tracked each year. Since the sinking of the *Titanic* there has not been a single ship-iceberg collision for vessels that have heeded the Ice Patrol's published limits of all known ice.

LESSON: If you can't eliminate the hazard, avoid it.

5.2. *Hurricane Warnings*

In 1900, with little warning, a hurricane hit Galveston, Texas, killing as many as eight thousand people, the worst loss of life from a natural disaster in U.S. history. Since then, weather forecasting has improved dramatically as a result of research and technological improvements such as radar, satellites, and computers. The National Weather Service is now able to provide warning days before a hurricane nears land. In the past the large majority of hurricane deaths were from the coastal storm surge. People now have time to evacuate the coast and go to safer locales. Currently, most hurricane deaths in the United States are due to inland flooding, when people who try to drive through moving water are at high risk for drowning.

From 1901 to 1930 approximately 130 people in the United States died each year from hurricanes; from 1931 to 1970 the average yearly death toll was 70. From 1971 to 2000, although about 40 million more Americans were living in coastal counties, the number of hurricane-related deaths fell to approximately 20 per year. According to the authors of the book *Hurricane Watch*:

> Without a doubt, the biggest success story of computer modeling and response has been the almost complete elimination of deaths from storm surge in the United States. From the beginning of good hurricane records through Hurricane Camille in 1969, storm surge was the leading hurricane killer in the United States. There's no question about this. But from Camille through the year 2000, storm surge took only five lives in the United States. . . . However, the threat remains large in vulnerable, densely populated area such as New Orleans . . . where even the best warning won't give people time to escape. Among the experts, the vulnerability of New Orleans is legendary and scary because a large part of the city and its suburbs are below sea level. (Sheets & Williams 2001, 214)

LESSON: Actions by many government agencies can help reduce injury, but there is still danger.

5.3. *Volcano Evacuation*

On the island of Luzon in the Philippines lies Mount Pinatubo, a volcano dormant for five hundred years. Through most of the twentieth century the mountain was inconspicuous, covered in dense rain forest; only about six hundred yards above the nearby plains, it is not clear that most people in the area even knew it was a volcano.

In mid-June 1991 Mount Pinatubo erupted, bringing total darkness to much of central Luzon. Ash was ejected to heights of over twenty miles. The eruption was one of the two largest in the twentieth century, ten times larger than the 1980 eruption of Mount St. Helens. Global effects were substantial. The injection of 17 million tons of sulfur dioxide into the atmosphere, the largest volume ever recorded by modern instruments, led to a decrease in global temperatures of 0.7 degrees Fahrenheit. The eruption also caused a substantial reduction in world ozone levels.

Fortunately scientists from the Philippine Institute of Volcanology and Seismology and the U.S. Geological Survey had forecast the eruption. In March and April a series of small earthquakes at Mount Pinatubo indicated that some kind of volcanic activity was imminent. Scientists immediately installed monitoring equipment and analyzed the volcano for clues to its previous eruptive history. Radiocarbon dating of charcoal found in old volcanic deposits revealed three major explosive eruptions, about 5,500, 3,500, and 500 years earlier.

Using the scientific information, civil and military leaders were able to order massive evacuations and take measures to protect property before the eruption. Between April and mid-June more than sixty-five thousand people left the area within twenty miles of the volcano. When the explosions occurred hundreds rather than tens of thousands of villagers died. The warnings and formal evacuations are credited with saving thousands of lives and hundreds of millions of dollars in property. Unfortunately the mudflows left sixty thousand people homeless.

LESSON: Don't fool with Mother Nature.

5.4. Tsunami Escape

In 1907 a tsunami caused by a huge earthquake hit the Simeulue community in Indonesia, killing a large number of its inhabitants. Many died when the ocean initially receded, exposing fish and coral. The inhabitants ran to the beach to collect the fish, not realizing that the water would come back—with a vengeance.

The Simeulue survivors made sure their children and grandchildren would learn from this tragedy. Infants were raised with lullabies of the tsunami. Through the island's oral history, children were taught what to do in an earthquake: wait to see if there are signs of a tsunami and, if there are, make quickly for the hills.

On December 26, 2004, Simeulue became the first coastline in the world to experience the terrible force of the great Indonesian tsunami, which killed over two hundred thousand people. Within ten minutes of the earthquake the sea receded some three hundred meters at the Simeulue coast; twenty minutes later the first tsunami wave arrived.

When the water began to be sucked out into the ocean, the Simeulue inhabitants raced to the hills, taking bicycles, motorbikes, and wheelbarrows piled with children. Only eight people out of the seventy-eight thousand island inhabitants died from the tsunami.

A high-tech tsunami detection system, such as the one already installed in the Pacific, would not have saved the islanders. The earthquake epicenter was only twenty-five miles away; by the time the warning sounded the waves would have already arrived.

In 2005 the United Nations Sasakawa Certificate of Merit was awarded to the Simeulue community for their diverse activities to build awareness about disaster risks. Simeulue is now cited as an example of the success of community-based disaster preparedness.

LESSON: We can learn injury prevention from the experiences of our
          grandparents.

5.5. Avalanche Transceivers

Snow avalanches are a natural process, occurring about a million times a year worldwide. Humans are sometimes caught in these avalanches. Between 1975 and 1995 the seventeen European and North and South American countries of the International Commission for Alpine Rescue averaged 146 avalanche fatalities per year. Interestingly, it is estimated that when people are caught in an avalanche, 95 percent of the time they or someone in their party triggered the slide.

Most avalanche victims die of asphyxiation from being buried in the snow. In the fifty-six avalanche deaths in Utah (1990–2006), 86 percent were due to asphyxiation; only 5 percent were due to trauma alone (e.g., hitting a tree; McIntosh et al. 2007).

Air pockets in the snow typically provide a few minutes of oxygen to the buried victim, hence time is the most critical issue during rescue. Estimated survival chances fall rapidly with time, from over 90 percent for a burial less than 15 minutes, to 30 percent after 35 minutes, to 3 percent after 130 minutes (Michahelles et al. 2003).

Rescue procedures entail three steps: localizing the victim, extricating the victim (typically with shovels), and providing first aid (e.g., opening respiratory tracts and avoiding hypothermia). The avalanche transceiver has become the key tool for step one: finding the victim quickly enough to save a life. The device does not prevent burial in an avalanche but is designed to reduce the amount of time one is buried.

The first effective avalanche transceiver was developed at Cornell Aeronautical Laboratory in 1968, and the first units were sold commercially in 1971. When turned on, the typical transceiver transmits an electronic beep; others in the party turn their beacon to receive, and the beep gets stronger the closer you get.

The receivers save lives. A study of buried avalanche victims in Austria found that having a transceiver was associated with a substantial reduction in median burial time (100 minutes without a transceiver to 20 minutes with a transceiver) and a 14 percent reduction in mortality (Hohlrieder et al. 2005). A study of U.S. avalanche victims found that 32 percent of buried victims without beacons survived, compared to 44 percent with beacons (McCammon & Hageli 2007). A study of larger avalanches in Canada found that 13 percent of buried victims without beacons survived, compared to 32 percent of those with beacons (Jamieson 1994).

Although these beacons help, they are clearly not a panacea. One problem is that practice and training are needed to locate victims quickly and dig them out (Atkins 1998).

Still, the beacons are a success story. They can save lives, and more and more people at risk are using them. A study in Utah during the 2006 winter season found that over 98 percent of backcountry skiers in Utah were carrying both avalanche transceivers and shovels; unfortunately, snowmobilers and snowshoers were much less prepared (Silverton et al. 2007).

> LESSON: Technology can reduce the likelihood of serious injury
> postevent as well as pre-event.

HEROES

5.a. Benjamin Franklin (1706–1790)

Benjamin Franklin was widely beloved, esteemed, and celebrated as the most famous scientist alive. "His name was familiar to government and people, to kings, courtiers, nobility, clergy, and philosophers, as well as plebeians, to such a degree that there was scarcely a peasant or a citizen, a valet de chambre, coachman or footman, a lady's chambermaid or a scullion in a kitchen, who was not familiar with it, and did not consider him as a friend to human kind" (Adams 1856, 660). Franklin's scientific fame continues today: his work on electricity is "recognized as ushering in a scientific revolution comparable to those wrought by Newton in the previous century or by Watson and Crick in ours" (Herschbach, cited in Isaacson 2003, 129).

Franklin's electrical theory, the conservation of charge, "must be considered to be of the same fundamental importance to physical science as Newton's law of conservation of momentum" (Isaacson 2003, 135). Franklin also came up with the distinction between insulators and conductors, the concepts of capacitors and batteries, and the idea of electrical grounding. "He found electricity a curiosity and left it a science" (Van Doren, cited in Isaacson 2003, 144).

Franklin first discussed his theories about lightning in 1749. In his lab he used a needle to draw off the charge of an iron ball. He believed that lofty towers, spires, and ships' masts similarly drew the fire from electrified clouds. His idea was to use a tall metal rod to draw some of the electric charge from the cloud. These "lightning rods" could be used to tame one of the greatest natural dangers. Franklin's letters were published and translated into French, and the French successfully tested his ideas. By 1752 he had become an international sensation, not only the most celebrated scientist in Europe and America, but a popular hero. By solving a great natural mystery he had conquered one of nature's most terrifying dangers.

In the early eighteenth century most New Englanders still lived in an "enchanted universe," a place of "dark impenetrable forces, vengeful thunderstorms, portentous comets, witches and ghosts. A belief in providential events and omens was common, as was the idea that an ongoing battle between Satan and God ruled many features of daily life" (Dray 2005, 7). It was generally believed that "what the people suffered was caused by their sins and that repentance alone could relieve them (historian Perry Miller, cited in Dray 2005, 16). By contrast, Franklin believed that salvation was to be achieved not through prayer, but by leading a virtuous life and helping others—that on Judgment Day we shall be examined not on what we thought, but on what we did.

Fortunately, by the mid-1700s an interest in science had become fashionable, one of the distinguishing characteristics of a gentleman. Enlightened minds had come to believe that science should be based on empirical findings and were confident that such an approach to science would lead to inventions that could improve well-being. The Franklin lightning rod represented a glorious example. Not surprisingly, the lightning rod met fierce religious resistance. The notion that man might tame the lightning was considered heretical, "an impious attempt to rob the Almighty of his thunder, to wrest the Bolt of Vengeance out of his Hand" (Dray 2005, 111). In 1755 Boston clergy accused Franklin of being responsible for a New England earthquake, claiming that his lightning rods had merely deflected heaven's resentment into the ground.

In France Franklin's ideas met fierce opposition from a clergyman-scientist, Abbé Nollet. As a churchman Nollet deemed it "as impious to ward off Heaven's lightning as for a child to ward off the chastening rod of its father" (quoted in Dray 2005, 96). As a scientist he rejected the suggestion that a slim iron rod placed on a rooftop could conquer the overwhelming power of a thunderstorm (Dray 2005).

An authoritative church history of Britain states that before lightning rods, "there was scarce a great abbey in England which was not burnt down with lightning from heaven" (quoted in Dray 2005, 67). In many localities, consecrated church bells would be rung at the approach of a storm to repel the demons and avert the lightning. This did not work. In Germany in a thirty-five year period in the mid-1770s close to four hundred churches were hit by lightning, and more than one hundred bell ringers were killed. In Venice, some three thousand people were killed when lightning hit a church where gunpowder had been stored to keep it safe—under God's protection.

"Few scientific discoveries have been of such immediate service to humanity" as the lightning rod (Isaacson 2003, 145). Not only did it save many lives and much property, but Franklin actually saved his own home. While he was abroad a bolt of lightning melted the tip of his lightning rod but spared his house, "so that at length," he wrote, "the invention has been of some use to the inventor" (quoted in Isaacson 2003, 441).

Franklin's forays in science were numerous. He invented bifocals and the Franklin stove. In the public health field alone he was one of the first to argue that cold and flu may be spread by contagion rather than cold air. He observed that people often catch cold from one another when shut up together in a close room. One way to prevent colds, he argued, was regular exercise. Franklin also correctly diagnosed that it was lead poisoning that caused much of the illness in painters, glazers, and plumbers. He learned that people who drank rum from stills that used metal coils often had similar symptoms and suggested that the coils be made of tin rather than of pewter, which contains lead.

But it was as the inventor of the lightning rod in which Franklin's scientific fame resided. This, along with his role in the American Revolution, led to the famous epigram in 1776 by the celebrated French economist Anne-Robert Jacques Turgo that captures Franklin's legacy: "He snatched lightning from the sky and the scepter from tyrants." "The lightning rod was one of the Enlightenment's greatest inventions not only for the lives and property it saved, but for its potent symbolism. . . . If reason can vanquish thunderbolts, can it also influence morality, social organization and human behavior?" (Dray 2005, 184).

5.b. William Redfield (1789–1857)

Hurricanes in the United States primarily come from across the West Atlantic, often striking through the Caribbean Sea and the Gulf of Mexico. When Columbus arrived in the Americas in 1492 he heard the native inhabitants speak fearfully of the storm god called Jurakan. On his fourth visit to the new world, a *jurakan* hit the Caribbean. His ships survived, but some twenty-five other vessels launched by the governor of Hispaniola foundered in the storm.

It is estimated that hurricanes have killed up to half a million people in the Western Hemisphere, most of these deaths occurring before the nineteenth century. In 1780, for example, some twenty-two thousand people lost their lives to hurricanes; at least half of these were sailors aboard ships.

Before the nineteenth century people had no real understanding of what storms were. Most believed that storms were chaotic maelstroms, whose winds shifted directions willy-nilly. Even the greatest storms were thought to develop and dissipate as acts of God.

On October 22, 1743, Benjamin Franklin in Philadelphia was planning to view the eclipse of the moon. But a storm hit Philadelphia, with the wind from the northeast. Franklin naturally assumed that the storm had come from Boston, also blocking the view of his friends there. Weeks later he discovered that the Bostonians had seen the eclipse, and that the storm had hit there early the next morning. He recognized that the storm—which was actually a hurricane—must not have traveled in the same direction as the wind.

However, it was not until 1831, when a self-taught American scientist, William Redfield, published an article in the *American Journal of Science* titled "On the Prevailing Storms of the Atlantic Coast," that the nature of hurricanes was revealed. The paper codified what meteorologists now call "the law of storms." The law gave sea captains, for the first time, some practical advice on how to maneuver their ships to increase the likelihood of surviving a hurricane.

Redfield collected and described in detail the patterns of damage from a storm that had hit New England ten years earlier. In one area of Connecticut the winds had blown a hundred miles per hour in a southwest direction. However, just forty miles north, in another part of Connecticut, the winds were blowing at about the same time in the opposite direction. Redfield showed that the winds were circulating around a calm center and how the storm had moved.

He concluded that "all violent gales or hurricanes are great whirlwinds, in which the wind blows in circuits around an axis; that the winds do not move in horizontal circles but rather in spirals; that the velocity of rotation increases from the margin toward the center of the storm; that the whole body of air is, at the same time, moving forward in a path, at a variable rate, but always with a velocity much less than its velocity of rotation" (quoted in Sheets & Williams 2001, 24).

Redfield had unlocked the secret of hurricanes with his "law of storms." He did not actually understand why hurricanes behave as whirlwinds (e.g., due to the influence of the rising heat and the spinning earth), but his inductive analysis correctly described their movements.

Redfield, an industrialist with a railroad and steamship business, was an amateur scientist who also conducted geological research, including original work on fish fossils. In 1848 he helped found the American Association for the Advancement of Science and served as the organization's first president. But his major accomplishment was in helping to reduce the loss of life in storms. Commodore Matthew Perry, who opened Japan to the West in 1853, wrote that seamen are indebted to Redfield "for the discovery of a law which has already contributed, and will continue to contribute, greatly to the safety of vessels traversing the ocean" (quoted in Sheets & Williams 2001, 25–26).

Denison Olmstead, a leading scientist of the time, in his memorial tribute to Redfield wrote, "In no department perhaps of the studies of nature [has] mankind been more surprised to find things governed by fixed laws than in the case of winds. . . . The researches of the meteorologists of our time force on us the conclusion that winds even in the violent forms of hurricanes . . . are governed by laws hardly less determinate than those which control the movements of the planets" (quoted in Sheets & Williams 2001, 29–30).

Olmstead wrote that as soon as Redfield had established that storms are whirlwinds, he "commenced that inquiry . . . to promote the safety of the immense amount of human life and of property that are afloat on the ocean and exposed continually to the dangers of shipwreck." Olmstead compared this contribution to Ben Franklin's work with lightning rods: "As every building saved from the ravages of lightning by the conducting rod is a token both of the sagacity and the benevolence of Franklin, so every vessel saved from the horrors of shipwreck by rules derived from these laws of storms, is a witness to the sagacity and benevolence of Redfield" (quoted in Sheets & Williams 2001, 26).

CHAPTER 6

Violence

INTRODUCTION

Intentional injury can be self-inflicted (e.g., suicide) or other-inflicted (e.g., homicide). In 2005, there were over 18,000 homicides in the United States and more than 32,000 suicides. The instrument in the majority of both homicides and suicides was a firearm. Intentional injury deaths accounted for almost 30 percent of total injury deaths in 2005. The CDC reported over 2 million nonfatal violence-related injuries for 2005; more than 80 percent of these were other-inflicted. Intentional injuries accounted for only 7 percent of nonfatal injuries seen in hospital emergency departments.

The World Health Organization divides other-inflicted violence into two parts: interpersonal and collective. Collective violence refers to incidents in which people who, identifying themselves as members of a group, use violence against another group or set of individuals in order to achieve political, economic, or social objectives. Collective violence includes war and the 9/11 terrorist attacks.

The distinction between intentional and unintentional injury is not always clear-cut. For example, if a burglar unexpectedly comes upon a resident and pushes him out of the way in order to flee the scene, any resulting injury is intentional. But if a motorist is intentionally speeding, or intentionally runs a red light, and causes a crash, the resulting injuries are usually classified as unintentional.

Like intentional injuries, unintentional injury can also be divided into self-inflicted or other-inflicted. You can close a door on your own hand, or someone else can close a door on your hand. You can dive into too shallow water and become injured, or someone can dive on top of you while you are in the water.

Intentional injuries are a subset of violent acts, some of which may cause harm to property or result in psychological intimidation. Unlike most unintentional injuries, violence may lead to much fear and social disruption; contrast the expected effects on the psyche of a small community of four fatal car crashes compared with four separate street murders.

There seem to be fewer clear intentional injury success stories compared with unintentional injury successes. Criminologists whom I asked could not readily give me examples of either successes or heroes of intentional violence prevention. There have been many policies designed to reduce violence, some of which seem to have been effective, such as certain school-based programs to reduce bullying, interventions to limit youth violence, and emergency department–based violence prevention programs (e.g., Vreeman & Carroll 2007; Limbos et al. 2007; Zun et al. 2006). Unfortunately even the successful interventions have typically been implemented at only one or two sites and have not been rolled out to or shown to be effective in other communities. They should be considered current "best practices" rather than success stories.

The success stories in this section examine both self-inflicted and other-inflicted injuries. The first three are self-inflicted, resulting in suicide. The first describes a comprehensive approach to reduce suicide in the U.S. Air Force, an approach touted as a model for other occupations. The second success story deals with reducing a risk factor not only for suicide, but for virtually all injuries: alcohol. By making alcohol less available, many suicides and other injuries were prevented.

The third story deals with the elimination in Britain of the availability of the most common means of suicide, carbon monoxide poisoning, which reduced not only carbon monoxide suicides but also total suicides. Either many suicidal people decided not to attempt suicide, or they used a less lethal alternative. The implication of this success story for other areas of intentional injury, specifically crime and violence, has been noticed. Blocking easy opportunities, even for individuals motivated to commit intentional injury, can help reduce overall levels of violence. Criminal activity will not be merely displaced if some targets of crime are made more impregnable (Clarke & Mayhew 1988).

The next three success stories deal directly with other-inflicted injuries, in the form of assaults. The first of these concerns the Washington, DC, Metro, which was an attempt to build a crime-free subway system. There was no attempt to change human nature—to make people better—but instead simply to make it more difficult to rob or assault another person, and thus make the system safer. Safety seems to build on itself; it is self-reinforcing. When people feel safe on the subway, more people ride the subway, making it even safer.

The architecture of the DC Metro is an illustration of "situational crime prevention," which focuses on changing the circumstances giving rise to crime rather than focusing on trying to detect and sanction offenders. More specifically, the case is an example of "crime prevention through environmental design" (CPTED). Examples of crime successes from the 1970s using the broad principles of CPTED include the virtual elimination of robberies of bus drivers in the United States by the creation of exact fare systems (i.e., the drivers had no money to steal) and the reduction in muggings in the London Underground due to the introduction of TV surveillance (Clarke & Mayhew 1980).

The next success story is also an illustration of situational crime prevention (pre-event). It tells of community-based efforts in four large tourist resort towns in Australia to reduce alcohol-related violence inside and outside of bars and nightclubs. Largely by inducing changes in managerial practices at these venues, community action helped improve the nightclub experience for patrons and reduced the crime too often associated with young males consuming alcohol.

The final success story in this chapter deals with the second row of the Haddon matrix: making the individual safer during the event. Police body armor doesn't seem to reduce attacks on police, but it makes it far less likely that police officers will be seriously injured, particularly in a shooting incident.

One of the models in Section 8 also deals with violence prevention. In that instance a comprehensive and innovative criminal justice approach, combined with community involvement, led to a large reduction in the most serious of violent injuries in the United States: firearm injuries. Unfortunately there have been not been enough indisputable success stories in the firearm injury area, at least in the United States (see chapter 9).

VIOLENCE SUCCESS STORIES

6.1. Suicide in the Air Force

Please go the extra mile to foster a sense of belonging.
Make sure your people feel they are a member of the

team at unit functions and other small gatherings. It
has been repeatedly demonstrated that social
connections save lives. . . . Let's ensure we take care of
our own—our Air Force family.

> —General Michael E. Ryan, *U.S. Air Force chief*
> *of staff, July 1999*

In the mid-1990s, suicide was the second leading killer of U.S. Air Force personnel, responsible for 24 percent of all deaths. Problems with relationships, finances, or the law played a part in the overwhelming majority of the suicides; fewer than one-third of the victims had accessed Air Force mental health services before their deaths..

With strong and visible support of the chief of staff, the Air Force created a population-based prevention program. The program was aimed at decreasing the stigma associated with seeking help for social or psychological problems, improving social networks, and enhancing understanding of mental health in the Air Force community. Features of the program included the message that it was not only acceptable, but a sign of strength, to recognize life problems and get professional help, and the message "We are not just another big corporation—we are the United States Air Force, and we 'take care of our own.'" In a 1999 survey almost three-quarters of Air Force unit commanders identified risk of suicide as their highest concern regarding behavioral health in their units.

The program was fully implemented in 1997. Suicide in the Air Force fell from a peak annual rate of 16.4 suicides per 100,000 (over 50 suicides) in 1994 to a trough of 3.5 per 100,000 in 1999. Comparing the 1990–1996 period to the 1997–2002 period, the suicide rate fell 33 percent. The program was also associated with a pronounced reduction in family violence and homicide. The Air Force approach was highlighted in an Institute of Medicine report in 2002 and suggested as a model for other occupational-related communities, such as law enforcement.

LESSON: A strong commitment from top leaders is often crucial for
          reducing injuries.

6.2. Suicide and Perestroika

Alcohol use is a risk factor for violent death, including suicide. The Soviet Union historically had a very serious alcohol problem, particularly among men. On June 1, 1985, Mikhail Gorbachev introduced a major antialcohol campaign in the USSR. The campaign included a decrease in alcohol production and in the number of retail outlets for alcohol; the quantity of alcohol sold was limited to half a liter of alcohol per person monthly; the price of alcohol was raised 80 percent; and police patrols were reinforced and empowered to issue fines or arrest people found drunk in public places. If alcohol was consumed at work, the person in charge could lose his or her job; workers showing any sign of having consumed alcohol could be fired. Representatives of state authorities were urged not to drink alcohol toasts during public receptions. For individuals to succeed socially, it became useful to belong to an abstainers' club; institutions were compelled to organize such clubs, whose activities were sponsored by the government. State TV promulgated the antialcohol message.

Alcohol consumption plummeted in all fifteen Soviet republics; for example, consumption fell over 50 percent in Russia in 1986 compared with 1984. Suicides, and male suicides in particular, also fell dramatically in every USSR republic. Male suicides in Russia fell 44 percent.

Several natural experiments—such as Prohibition in the United States, sharply increased alcohol prices in Denmark (1911–1924), and restrictions on the sale of alcohol in Sweden in connection with the introduction of ration books in the 1950s—have been associated with substantial decreases in suicide rates. However, perestroika has been reasonably called "history's most effective suicide preventive program for men" (Wasserman 2001, 254). How much the drop in suicide was due to hope of a better future, greater freedom, or the strict alcohol policy is unknown, but the decreased rate of suicides, and of all violent deaths, was dramatic.

> LESSON: Alcohol is a risk factor for both unintentional and
>   intentional injury; reducing alcohol consumption can help
>   reduce injury.

6.3. Gas Suicide in Britain

In 1963 suicide by domestic gas (putting one's head in the oven) accounted for 41 percent of all completed suicides in England and Wales. As a method of suicide, carbon monoxide (CO) poisoning had many advantages. The gas was widely available (in 80 percent of British homes), and the method required little planning or specialized knowledge. Death was painless, did not result in disfigurement, and did not produce a mess; there was no blood. Death typically occurred within half an hour; most victims were discovered dead.

TABLE 3

Suicide in England and Wales

Year	Gas Suicides (number)	Gas Suicides (rate per 100,000)	Non-Gas Suicides (number)	Non-Gas Suicides (rate per 100,000)	Total Suicides (number)	Total Suicides (rate per 100,000)
1963	2,368	5.0	3,346	7.1	5,714	12.2
1975	23	0.0	3,670	7.5	3,693	7.5

SOURCE: Clarke R.V., Mayhew P. 1988. The British gas suicide story and its criminological implications. *Crime and Justice* 10:88.

In the late 1950s new gas manufacturing technology began to be introduced in Britain, lowering the CO content of the gas. A larger change occurred between 1968 and the mid-1970s with the conversion of the British gas supply to North Sea gas, which is free of carbon monoxide. Between 1963 and 1975, the average CO content in British domestic gas fell from 10.7 to 0 percent.

Suicide by gas poisoning also fell dramatically. In 1963 2,368 domestic gas suicides were recorded in England and Wales. That number fell to 23 in 1975. Most important, non-gas suicide death rates remained largely unchanged, resulting in over two thousand fewer total suicides. This occurred during a period when the unemployment rate in Britain rose 50 percent, traditionally a time when suicide rates increase.

Although not designed or promoted as a suicide prevention policy, the removal of carbon monoxide from the British gas supply may be considered the most effective such policy in British history (Table 3).

LESSON: Unintended consequences can be beneficial as well as detrimental.

6.4. Washington, DC, Metro

The Washington, DC, subway system, the Metro, which opened in 1976, is specifically designed to deter criminals and make riders feel comfortable and secure. A high level of natural surveillance is achieved through having high, freestanding vaulted ceilings, with a minimal number of supporting columns that could provide cover for criminals. Long, winding corridors and corners found in many older systems are deliberately avoided. Lighting is recessed to avoid shadows. There are no public restrooms, luggage lockers, excess chairs and benches, or fast-food facilities, so that potential offenders are not encouraged to linger. The system is closed during low-density early morning hours.

All stations have at least eight strategically placed closed-circuit TV cameras. Trains are characterized by a straight-through design, enabling police to walk freely between cars. Each car has passenger-to-operator intercoms. Station attendants carry two-way radios.

These and many other measures were created specifically to keep the Metro crime rate low. And they have succeeded. Washington, DC, subway crime (e.g., murder, rape, robbery, assault) is typically 75 percent lower than the rates seen in the subway systems of Atlanta, Chicago, or Boston.

LESSON: Design and management plans that make it harder to
          offend can prevent violence and other crimes from
          occurring.

6.5. Nightclub Violence

Surfers Paradise is a large tourist resort in Queensland, Australia. In the early 1990s it had more than 250,000 permanent residents and each year attracted millions of visitors. At that time there were twenty-two nightclubs in the small central business district.

A major problem in the early 1990s was the large amount of violence and disorder in the central business district in the early morning hours, as hundreds of drunken revelers emerged from the nightclubs. Not only was the community enraged, but the businesses were losing money because of the area's poor reputation, and a $4 billion tourist industry was threatened by international reports of violence against tourists.

To reduce the alcohol-related problems the city council provided some funds for a community initiative. A steering committee was formed and a project officer hired. Training was provided to bar bouncers and for improved relations between the police and these private security personnel.

A key to the success of the program was the creation of a task force designed to improve bar management in these nightclubs. For the first time the bar owners were involved in a positive process of problem identification in the community and asked to contribute to the solution. Each was asked to help create and publicize a Code of Practice concerning the delivery of alcohol in a responsible manner. A committee of their peers and other business leaders were charged with monitoring whether the bars adhered to the code.

Within a few months venue managers had employed more security guards and helped increase the availability of taxis after hours. Trained university students acting as unobtrusive patron-observers reported that the bouncers were friendlier and the bars and rest rooms were cleaner. Food was more readily available. There were fewer drink promotions. The patrons seemed more relaxed. There was less drunkenness, swearing, and rowdiness and less blatant sexual activity. Verbal abuse declined 82 percent, arguments 68 percent, and physical assaults 52 percent. "The impact of the Code of Practice was particularly apparent, with substantial improvements in responsible hospitality practices and consequent reductions in levels of aggression and violence" (Homel et al. 1997, 70).

In the following years this problem-focused community safety approach was replicated in three additional Queensland resort cities: Cairns, Townsville, and Mackay. Again a key feature was to encourage nightclub managers to introduce a Code of Practice covering security staff, alcohol promotions, and alcohol use. The goal was to help create comfortable surroundings that do not frustrate patrons, to engage in practices that discourage drinking to intoxication and foster a positive social atmosphere, and to create clear rules and limits that would be enforced by well-trained and peace-loving bar workers and security staff.

In nightclubs at these locations lighting improved, as did the cleanliness of toilets and the availability of taxis and public transport. Decorum expectations of management increased, so the venues became less permissive, especially in terms of overt risqué sexual activity (while flirtatious "checking out" and "chatting up" increased). There was a reduction in the use of promotions that encourage rapid alcohol consumption. More food was available. A friendlier bar and security staff had a better focus on controlling risky features of the environment. There was a marked decline in the incidence of high levels of male intoxication and a drop in rowdiness, swearing, and group territoriality. The overall level of sociability, cheerfulness, and friendliness was rated much higher (especially for women). These changes appeared good for business. Patronage and crowding increased, and average drinking rates remained unchanged.

In terms of violence, results were also astounding. Verbal abuse fell 60 percent in the bars in these cities, challenges and threats fell 40 percent, and physical assaults dropped more than 75 percent.

LESSON: It is possible to make small alterations to a drinking
                 environment to dramatically change the level of violence.

6.6. Police Body Armor

To protect themselves from injury in combat and other dangerous situations, throughout history humans have used various materials, from animal skins, to wood, to metal, to fabric. Soft armor, made of silk, was first explored by the military in the late nineteenth century but was effective only against low-velocity bullets. During World War II the "flak jacket," constructed of nylon, provided protection from munitions fragments but was not effective against most pistols or rifles.

From 1966 to 1971 the annual number of law enforcement officers killed in the line of duty in the United States rose from 57 to 129. Recognizing that most of the fatalities were inflicted with handguns, the predecessor to the National Institute of Justice (NIJ) instituted a research program to develop lightweight body armor that police could wear full time. Working with private contractors (e.g., the Aerospace firm MITRE Corporation) and other government agencies (the National Bureau of Standards, the U.S. Army, the FBI) the program developed effective, lightweight body armor using DuPont's Kevlar fabric, which had been developed to replace steel belting in vehicle tires. The research program helped solve many of the initial problems of Kevlar, for example, that its penetration resistance was degraded when wet and by sunlight, washing, and dry cleaning. By the mid-1970s body armor was commercially available. In 2001 more than eighty manufacturers were producing body armor and participating in the NIJ's voluntary compliance testing program.

Between 1973 and 2001 over twenty-five hundred "saves" were attributed to the use of body armor, most during felonious assaults but a substantial minority during accidents such as car crashes. A case-control study found that among officers shot in the upper torso, 75 percent of those without body armor died compared to 18 percent who were wearing body armor. Between 1992 and 2001 no officer died from a handgun round that penetrated his or her body armor; nineteen did die in incidents involving rifle rounds that their armor could not withstand.

Although the number of police more than doubled between the mid-1970s and 2000, the annual number of officer homicides fell from over 120 in the early 1970s to slightly over 40 by the last years of the twentieth century.

> LESSON: A concerted effort by private organizations and
>   government agencies can have life-saving results.

HEROES

6.a. Thomas Mott Osborne (1859–1926)

Thomas Mott Osborne, known as "the pioneer and prophet of prison reform" ("The Osborne Family" 2008), was born into a progressive political family. His great-aunt and grandmother organized the world's first women's rights conference in 1848. His aunt married the son of the antislavery publisher William Lloyd Garrison. His feminist, antislavery mother was the unofficial guardian of Harriet Tubman.

At age 27 Thomas Osborne was made president of the DM Osborne company, the family's large farm machinery manufacturing business. In 1903 the family sold the company to International Harvester, leaving the 44-year-old Osborne with time and money to pursue his interests in social reform and public service. He founded and became the editor of his hometown newspaper in Auburn, New York, and was elected mayor of that city. At the state level, he was a vocal anti–Tammany Hall reformer.

In 1913 he was appointed by the governor of New York to chair a new commission on prison reform. Osborne decided to experience prison life and had himself incarcerated in the large Auburn prison under the name of Tom Brown. In prison clothing he shared the inmates' experiences. His experiment made front-page news, and his book *Within Prison Walls*, published in 1914, memorialized the event.

Osborne emerged from the week's confinement as America's most prominent crusader for improvement in prison conditions. He became determined to see American prisons transformed from "human scrap heaps into human repair shops." His major thesis was that prisoners must be treated as human to be human: "In prison, as elsewhere, when men are dominated by fear, brutality is the inevitable result" (quoted in Chamberlain 1935, 251).

At the prison in Auburn Osborne instituted a Mutual Welfare League composed of all the prisoners and based on the then novel principle of inmates' self-rule. The League was an attempt to train prisoners' in self-government and to prepare them to return to society. Osborne's program was modeled on a business contract: the prisoners were required to display better general discipline, a courteous attitude toward prison officers, cleanliness, and efficiency in work. In return they would be able largely to police themselves, which meant fewer guards and more privileges if the experiment succeeded.

And the experiment was a resounding success. Inmates knew they were all responsible for the success of the League, and misbehavior of any of the men would jeopardize the entire experiment. The League eliminated the terrible rule of silence, according to which inmates were not allowed to talk to each other; it also expanded outdoor recreation, instituted weekly movies and entertainments, formed a band, and organized vocational and educational programs. In return, order increased and violence decreased.

For minor crimes committed while in prison the main penalty imposed by the League itself was suspension from the League, and with it the privileges of membership. In the past a man disciplined by prison authorities was a hero and there was a certain glory in martyrdom. Now, when his own fellows deemed him unworthy of participating in their organization, he became an outcast.

The League also assisted discharged prisoners. In addition to providing food and clothing, the League was a support organization to help bridge the gap between incarceration and freedom with vocational placement and counseling.

In 1914 Osborne was appointed warden of Sing Sing Prison in Ossining, New York. His experiment in prisoner self-government there was also a marked success. The Prisoners' Court, run by the inmates, dealt with all crimes. Immediate reforms of Sing Sing's Mutual Welfare League included allowing visitors on Sundays and holidays, permitting the inmates to buy postage stamps, and leaving lights on a half-hour later for reading.

Inmate insubordination, dope smuggling, and violent crime became rare as the prisoners policed themselves. The inmates knew that everyone would suffer if violent crime erupted and anyone escaped. In 1915 the League leaders appealed to the inmates to relinquish all weapons, and 150 knives were turned in. In 1914 more than 372 emergency cases (mostly violence-related) had to be treated at the prison hospital, close to 25 percent of the total population of prisoners; after the League was instituted in 1915, despite more prisoners the number had decreased to 86.

Critics denounced Osborne's reforms as a system for coddling criminals. His time at Sing Sing was marred by trumped-up charges of malfeasance and even immorality from Tammany and other enemies. The defense of Osborne included a letter signed by a hundred guards stating "most emphatically," "Never in the history of this prison have such cordial and kindly relations been established and maintained between the Warden, the inmates, and ourselves" (quoted in Chamberlain 1935, 349). The judge of the court that sentenced the majority of Sing Sing felons wrote, "The proof of the pudding is in the

eating. Since Mr. Osborne undertook his noble work, I have not had
one man released from his supervision brought into my court" (quoted
in Chamberlain 1935, 396). When all charges against Osborne were
dropped more than forty ex-cons, members of the outside branch of
the Mutual Welfare League, came back to Sing Sing to celebrate his
vindication. However, Osborne was embittered by the political malice
he had encountered, and expecting more, in 1917 he resigned from
Sing Sing.

That year the secretary of the navy asked Osborne to go underground
again, this time at the Portsmouth Naval Prison in Kittery, Maine, then
known as the "Alcatraz of the East." Afterward Osborne headed the
prison, from 1917 to 1920, instituting numerous reforms, including
allowing outdoor recreation and forming a drama club. One mark of
his success was that more than four thousand able-bodied men from the
prison were able to return to service during the Great War. Osborne is
now known as the "Father of Naval Corrections" (Haasenritter 2003).

In the 1920s Osborne continued his personal inspections of prisons,
wrote books on prison reform, and "continued to be penology's most
potent weapon, a figure of international fame and influence" ("Thomas
Mott Osborne" 2002). After his death organizations he helped found—
the National Society of Penal Information and the Welfare League
Association—merged into the Osborne Association.

The Osborne Association continues to this day. With headquarters in
New York City, the Association currently has a paid staff of some 150,
many of them former prisoners. It operates a wide range of direct service programs, including specific programs focused on parenting, crack
addiction treatment, and HIV/AIDS services. The Association also continues to provide ex-prisoners with lodging, job information, and general social services that are calculated to help reduce recidivism. The
programs thus not only serve ex-prisoners but also the community by
reducing crime and violence.

6.b. Fathers Edward Flanagan (1886–1948) and Gregory Boyle (1954–)

In 1917 Father Edward J. Flanagan, a Roman Catholic priest, founded
America's most famous orphanage in Omaha, Nebraska, a place with
no fences, gates, locks, or bolts. The 1938 movie Boys Town, starring
Spencer Tracy as Father Flanagan, dramatized how this nonprofit,
nonsectarian organization provided the boys with a safe and loving

environment where they could gain the confidence and skills to become productive citizens.

Father Flanagan's goal was to make Boys Town a training place for good character: "It is not enough to see that what has been called an underprivileged child is given good food, warm clothing, and a clean bed. An army commissary can do as much. No! More than food, clothes, and shelter, what these lads have been deprived of is mother's tenderness, and father's wisdom, and the love of a family. We will never get anywhere in our reform schools and orphan asylums until we compensate for that great loss in such young lives" (quoted in Oursler & Oursler 1949, 5).

Father Flanagan's most famous phrase was "There is no such thing as a bad boy." He won numerous awards during his life. In 1999 readers of the *Daily Catholic* voted him one of the top one hundred Catholics of the twentieth century.

Boys Town is no longer just an orphanage, but a center for troubled youth. In 1979 it opened its arms to girls as well as boys. The Village of Boys Town, Inc., is an incorporated village in Nebraska, with seventy-six homes, a post office, fire and police departments, chapels, schools, and a working farm. It provides food, clothing, shelter, education, spiritual guidance, and medical care to abused, abandoned, and neglected children ages 9 to 19 from around the nation. A key is that the child must want to come to the village. Girls Town and Boys Town currently care for thousands of children and families each year in programs located at nineteen sites.

A Jesuit priest, Father Gregory Boyle, described as a "larger-than-life gospel-toting champion of (Los Angeles's) most despised and marginalized adolescents" (Fremon 1995, 8), also believes in the power of love to reform troubled teenagers. A probation officer once told him that he'd been in and out of Juvenile Hall as a kid, but that there was one person who never gave up on him. And that made all the difference. Boyle said, "It may sound simplistic, but I believe in that strategy with all my heart. A success for me is when it is clear to a kid that there exists at least one person who will love you no matter what. Most of us have tons of people in our lives who have that no-matter-what quality to the relationships. These kids don't. So hang on to your hat because their behavior will reflect that lack. And that's what this whole mess is about" (quoted in Fremon 1995, 18).

What does a barrio kid do when family and society have failed him? When he turns 14 or 15 he joins a gang, a surrogate family, where he finds loyalty, self-definition, discipline, even love. Father Boyle provides an alternative. "Whenever Greg's office door opens, gang members swoop in like baby chicks for a feeding. . . . The gangsters have rechristened Greg with his own *placa,* his street name: G-Dog. But most simply call him G" (Fremon 1995, 11).

Father Boyle's strategy for gangs is a three-pronged approach: prevention, intervention, and suppression. Prevention entails reaching kids when they are young and not yet in a gang; intervention includes providing better alternatives to those already in a gang; and suppression requires a strong police force to protect neighborhoods. Of the three, intervention has been the neglected stepchild, and Father Boyle's response has been to find jobs for former Los Angeles gang members. He created "Jobs for a Future/Homeboy Industries" to provide thousands of jobs, counseling, and other services (e.g., free tattoo removal) to former gang members who might otherwise be unemployable. Jobs for a Future creates opportunities so that at-risk youth "can plan their futures and not their funerals." A driving principle of Homeboy Industries is that "nothing stops a bullet like a job."

At-risk youth are placed in both external and internal jobs. Internal ventures include Homeboy Bakeries, which trains members from different gangs to become bakers, and Homeboy Silkscreen, which prints logos on apparel. Other ventures include Homeboy Landscaping and Homeboy Graffiti Removal. There is now a Homegirl Café.

It all started in 1988, when Father Boyle was the pastor at Dolores Mission, one of the poorest parishes in the city, nestled in two housing projects with eight very active warring gangs. There were shootings every night; between 1988 and 2004 Father Boyle buried 122 youth killed from gang violence.

Father Boyle's work has been inspirational and effective and has helped thousands of at-risk youth, which has helped reduce the number of killings. He says:

> I've never met a hopeful kid who joined a gang. . . . Any gang member is really coming from a place of misery that's kind of intense, you know, and a despair that's dark and bleak. And the bleaker it is, the more that kid's going to act out. And so I just think they find themselves unparented and drifting and gravitating perilously close to a gang and then they find themselves in it. And then, you know, before they know it, they have a record. And before they know it, it's been years since they've been formally educated. And then pretty soon it just becomes this dark place that you have to reach down and say, "Come on. You know, it's not a hole in the end. It's a tunnel. And trust me, there's light. And I'll walk with you till you get to the light. After such time, you can walk on your own." (Gross 2004)

Father Boyle has won numerous awards, including the 2000 California Peace Prize from the California Wellness Foundation and the 2001 Dignitas Humana Award from St. John's University.

6.c. Erin Pizzey (1939–)

Intimate partner violence is common in the United States, and throughout the world. A large national survey in the United States found that over 22 percent of women had been assaulted by an intimate partner (e.g., current or former spouse, cohabiting partner, boyfriend or girlfriend, or date) at least once in their lifetime. Each year in the United States more than a million women are physically assaulted by an intimate partner. Women are more at risk for violence from their intimate partner than from strangers or acquaintances: almost two-thirds of the women who report being raped, physically assaulted, and/or stalked since age 18 are victimized by an intimate partner (Tjaden & Thoennes 1998).

Violence against women was long an acceptable part of marriage. Indeed, it was not until 1871 that Alabama, and then Massachusetts, became the first states to rescind the legal right of men to beat their wives. In 1882 Maryland became the first state to make wife beating a crime. Still, in 1910 the U.S. Supreme Court denied a wife the right to prosecute her husband for assault because to do so "would open the doors of the courts to accusations of all sorts of one spouse against another." It was not until 1966 that beatings first became grounds for divorce in New York—but the plaintiff had to establish that a "sufficient" number of beatings had taken place.

The feminist movement of the 1960s and 1970s helped reverse the world's acceptance of intimate partner violence, especially violence against women. In 1971 Erin Pizzey recognized that many young mothers felt isolated, cut off in their homes. She opened a small community center where women and their children could come to meet and escape their loneliness. The center was a house that was open to any woman (men were allowed by invitation only), a place that was run and ruled by the women who stayed there. Chiswick Women's Aid quickly turned into a shelter for battered women.

At the time, homeless shelters in England were not sex segregated, and there was no place a women could go to escape a violent partner. The general policy of the British social services was to try not to interfere with the sanctity of marriage. Within two years, Chiswick Women's

Aid was getting a hundred telephone calls a day. "Women of all areas, classes and races were crying out for help as soon as they knew there was somebody who would listen and could do something to help them" (Pizzey 1977, 23). Pizzey soon had to find more houses for the women: "When space is made available, it is immediately taken up by people who badly need it" (Pizzey 1977, 46).

Chiswick Women's Aid received much publicity, including an article in 1974 in the European edition of *Time*, and the model was copied throughout the world. By 1996 there were over twelve hundred battered women's shelters in the United States alone.

In 1974 Pizzey also wrote the first book focusing on wife beating, *Scream Quietly or the Neighbors Will Hear*. The book was a landmark publication, helping to break the habit of secrecy that kept battered women from leaving home and seeking help. At the time, sociology courses on marriage and the family contained no reference to spousal abuse; the major emphasis was on female "adjustment" to marriage. Textbooks on social problems discussed violence, but violence in the streets, never in the home. From 1939 to 1970 the index to the *Journal of Marriage and the Family* did not include a reference to violence. Pizzey's small book helped open the closet door of domestic violence. A documentary of *Scream Quietly* was shown on PBS television in 1979.

Pizzey parted company with the women's movement in the 1970s owing to a difference in underlying philosophies. Although she describes herself as a feminist in *Scream Quietly*, she later became an ardent antifeminist. Pizzey came to believe that feminists were trying to destroy the family and that they would not recognize that many women themselves were violent.

Erin Pizzey has received various awards, including the International Order of Volunteering for Peace, Diploma of Honor (Italy) in 1981. She was a pioneer in providing help to battered women and in making intimate partner violence a public issue.

CHAPTER 7

Medical Treatment

INTRODUCTION

The last grid in the Haddon matrix (Cell 9), the environment/postevent, belongs largely to medical care and rehabilitation. Fortunately there have been dramatic improvements in these areas in the past two hundred years.

The development of trauma care has mirrored advances in surgery in general, benefiting from the introduction of anesthesia, antibiotics, aseptic techniques, imaging techniques, and other discoveries and inventions. Imaging techniques alone, including angiography, ultrasound, computed tomography (CT), and magnetic resonance imaging (MRI), developed since the end of the nineteenth century, have revolutionized both the accuracy of diagnoses and the treatment of trauma patients.

Throughout history weapons in warfare have become more destructive. Fortunately medical treatment for the wounded has also improved dramatically. Indeed, medical treatment has benefited tremendously from warfare; major advances specifically in the care of trauma victims have typically originated from the care of soldiers.

In the ancient world medicine reached its greatest heights in those societies that had no strongly established religious priesthood (e.g., Greece, Rome). It was in military medicine that physicians were most free from the strictures of religiously derived medical theory and where the best clinical medicine was practiced. For example, Egyptian military physicians developed effective treatment techniques for dealing with fractures of the skull, and Roman military doctors invented and used the tourniquet and arterial clamp (Gabriel & Metz 1992).

However, it is generally accepted that the true beginning of modern wound surgery occurred in 1545, with the publication of a book by Ambroise Pare, a military surgeon. Instead of the custom of pouring boiling oil into a wound to stop the putrefaction, Pare championed the idea of keeping medicaments out of wounds and allowing nature to perform its work. His motto was "I dressed him and God healed him." His rejection of cauterizing wounds and the introduction of the ligature to control hemorrhage should have revolutionized wound care. But, "like most steps forward, this was by no means accepted by the majority of surgeons" (Pruitt et al. 2003, 11).

During the Napoleonic era, France's Baron Larrey (1766–1842) emphasized the importance of surgical intervention before the anesthetic effect of the injury per se dissipated. He expanded the role of the military surgeon to include sanitation and food for the patients, training of medical personnel, and the transport of injured soldiers from the battlefield. He is best remembered as the pioneer of the horse-drawn "flying ambulances," which picked up the wounded as soon as possible and moved them rapidly to a position just behind the battle lines.

The advent of nursing care for the wounded occurred during the Crimean War (1853–1856). Florence Nightingale established food services, clean water, hospital laundry, bathrooms, and housekeeping and eventually championed sanitary improvements. This ministering angel also quickly became a national heroine.

Unfortunately, at the beginning of the American Civil War, one of the bloodiest wars ever fought, the lessons from these previous wars were ignored. The flying ambulance was nonexistent, as was systematic nursing care. In addition, "laudable pus" was still considered the goal of a healing wound, and ligatures applied to blood vessels were left hanging out of the wound. The major cause of death of the wounded soldier was infection secondary to surgery. Hospital gangrene and staphylococcal and streptococcal infections were rampant. Instruments were not sterilized, surgeons rarely washed their hands, and sponges used to clean out the pus of one wound were applied to the next without washing them. General anesthesia—America's great contribution to the medical world in the nineteenth century—introduced in 1847, was not put into more general use until after the war ended. Anesthesia helped in managing hemorrhage by allowing surgeons to perform a more deliberate operation.

As the Civil War progressed medical treatment improved. Union Army Surgeon General William Hammond began selecting medical directors for the field armies based on their competence rather than via the old boy network that stressed rank and connections (Greenwood & Berry 2005). He established a policy that only the three physicians in each division with the most extensive surgical experience would be permitted to perform surgical operations. That policy, which helped make demonstrated surgical expertise a requirement for receiving the title of "operating surgeon," has been identified "as one of the most momentous medical reforms to come out of the Civil War" (Rutkow 2005, 203).

In the nineteenth century rates of infection following surgery slowly began to decrease. France's Louis Pasteur discovered bacteria as the source of infection, and the British surgeon Joseph Lister developed a machine to spray carbolic acid in wounds. Although the mortality rate for Lister's patients dropped precipitously, his work was not immediately accepted; most surgeons thought it was nonsense to suggest that something that could not be seen was the cause of infection.

Ideas from Lister's work, including the steam sterilization of surgical materials and instruments, were used in Germany during the Franco-Prussian War (1870–1871), saving many lives. Still, although major advances were made in treating trauma in the nineteenth century, it was not until well into the twentieth century that a wounded soldier had a good chance of survival. For example, in the Franco-Prussian War an open fracture was generally regarded as a death sentence. Of over thirteen thousand amputations performed by French surgeons during that war, more than 75 percent of the soldiers died (Oliver 2001).

Both time to treatment and type of treatment of combat injuries improved dramatically in the twentieth century. The improvements in trauma care can be illustrated by the case-fatality rates from one type of war injury: abdominal wounds. In the Civil War there was an 87 percent mortality rate following abdominal wounds, which were always treated nonoperatively. In the Spanish American War mortality from abdominal wounds in the U.S. Army fell to 65 percent. World War I saw field ambulances for the first time that were motor-driven rather than horse-drawn. Abdominal wounds began being treated operatively, and blood transfusions were used to good advantage. The practice of closing all wounds was also stopped; in 1917 the Allies issued an edict that all war wounds should be left open. In World War I the mortality rate from abdominal wounds fell to 45 percent, but there was still no clear understanding of the cause of shock (Pruitt et al. 2003).

During World War II, wounded soldiers were evacuated by plane for the first time, and the importance of blood volume replacement after penetrating wounds became fully established. Antibiotics made wound infections much less of a problem. Wound cleansing, debridement, and immobilization of arm and leg fractures became standard procedures. Some medical historians believe that making debridement—the removal of devitalized tissue and foreign material from the wound—standard treatment was of paramount importance (Rich & Burris 2005). In World War II the mortality rate after abdominal wounds fell to 15 percent, although treating shock was still a problem.

During the Korean War increased understanding of the pathophysiology of injury and shock led to further advances. In the early years of the war, before the magnitude of blood loss in casualties was fully appreciated, there was evidence of renal failure in more than one-third of autopsied fatalities. After 1952 the prompt infusion of adequate volumes of resuscitation fluid reduced the occurrence of renal failure in those autopsied to under 1 percent (Pruitt 2006). In the Korean War the U.S. Army also introduced both the widespread use of helicopters and mobile army surgical hospital units to reduce the time to treatment. The mortality rate following abdominal wounds fell to 9 percent. In the Vietnam War advances in pulmonary treatment for shock helped further reduce the mortality rate from wounds in the U.S. Army.

Treatment of all types of wounds improved in the twentieth century. From the World War I to Vietnam surgical mortality for head wounds among U.S. Army personnel fell from 40 to 10 percent, for thorax wounds from 37 to 7 percent, and for abdominal wounds from 45 to 9 percent. Overall, mortality for wounded American soldiers fell from 8.1 percent in World War I, to 4.5 percent in World War II, to under 2.4 percent in Korea and 1.2 percent in Vietnam. The average transport time to treatment fell from 6 hours in World War I, to 5 hours in World War II, to 3 hours in Korea, to less than 1 hour in Vietnam (Foss 1989).

Reducing transport time to care has proved crucial for recovery from serious wounds. Although surgeons formerly talked of the "Golden Hour," during which most trauma victims could be saved if treatment was started, in our most recent wars injuries have been so severe that an hour wasn't fast enough. The U.S. Army therefore began using Forward Surgical Teams, traveling in Humvees directly behind the troops and right onto the battlefield. The speed of current surgical treatment of the wounded is largely responsible "for what we have seen in the current wars in Iraq and Afghanistan: a marked, indeed, historic reduction in the lethality of battle wounds" (Gawande 2007a, 53).

Unfortunately improvements in military care are often slow to reach civilians. In the United States in the 1960s "hospitals receiving trauma patients were ill-equipped and ill-staffed to handle injured patients and pre-hospital care consisted of poorly trained personnel with little equipment. During peak hours and at night these emergency rooms were often staffed with the most junior or unprepared physicians or poorly trained 'moonlighters.' In the ambulance, there was often only a driver with little emergency training" (Liberman et al. 2004). Indeed, it was not until the early 1960s that California became the first state with regulated and regionalized ambulance services.

The lack of systematic trauma care was highlighted in a 1966 National Academy of Sciences report, whose recommendations form the basis of trauma systems today. Among other things, the report highlighted many of the lessons learned on the battlefields in terms of triage, rapid transport of trauma patients, and improved prehospital care that could be applied effectively to civilian trauma patients.

The seriousness of any injury depends not only on the specific nature of the injury, but on the medical care and rehabilitation services available. The success stories in this chapter highlight a few of the many advances in medicine and rehabilitation that have helped reduce mortality, and the physical and social seriousness of injury. Although most advances were met with either initial indifference or outright hostility, the improvement in care over the past centuries has been phenomenal. The root causes of this remarkable, continual progress in science and medicine were the Enlightenment and the political revolutions that permitted the intellectual freedom "against dogmatism, charlatanism and metaphysics which before this time had restricted human thought" (Pruitt et al. 2003, 7).

Medical treatment continues to improve. Even in the twenty-first century many important low-tech improvements are still possible; they require only a willingness to change. For example, there is evidence that something as simple as a checklist (similar to a pilot's checklist) can substantially reduce medical errors. A five-item checklist to tackle the problem of line infections at one intensive care unit (ICU) reduced the ten-day line infection rate from 11 percent to zero, and the overall infection rate at multiple ICUs in Michigan fell some 66 percent (Gawande 2007b; Pronovost et al. 2006).

Indeed, simple changes are often the most effective. A few years ago a physician who had taken my injury prevention course sent me this email:

> There was an electrical incident in the cardiac operating room here caused by the circuits being overloaded. The room was rewired with more power and more outlets, but still when personnel plugged in equipment there were often overloads—they weren't using the right outlets for the various pieces

of equipment. What to do? I thought of the injury prevention course and suggested taking pictures of the equipment in the room and putting the photos at the outlet where each piece should be plugged in. This seemed to work, and they were impressed.

TREATMENT SUCCESS STORIES

7.1. Acute Care for Burn Injury

Over the past half-century major improvements have occurred in the treatment of burn patients. At the end of World War II, for example, *fewer* than half of the patients survived burns involving 40 percent of their total body-surface area. By the late 1990s *more than* half of all patients survived burns involving 80 percent of their total body-surface area. This remarkable success can be attributed to various therapeutic developments, including vigorous fluid resuscitation, early excision of burn wounds, advances in critical care and nutrition, prompt treatment of infection with powerful antibiotics, the development and use of effective skin substitutes, and the evolution of specialized burn centers.

Today almost all children with burn injuries on less than 60 percent of their body-surface area can be saved, and many with more massive burns can survive. Fortunately, although some children surviving very severe burns have lingering physical disability, most have a satisfying quality of life.

LESSON: Improving trauma care reduces injury fatality rates.

7.2. Trauma Systems

The creation of trauma systems helps ensure that patients are treated in the most appropriate facilities. Studies of trauma systems indicate that they reduce mortality by 15 to 20 percent for very seriously injured patients who are treated at trauma centers versus nontrauma centers.

A study of a trauma system in San Diego County found that, before the formal system, 32 percent of major trauma victims received suboptimal care, compared with 4 percent after the formal system was established. Preventable deaths occurred in 14 percent of fatalities before the implementation of the trauma system, compared with 3 percent after implementation.

Regional trauma care also saves on costs. Compared to states without regional systems, states with trauma care systems have 15 percent lower costs per hospitalized injury episode and 10 percent lower costs for nonhospitalized injury. In 1990 the federal government authorized a grants program to promote the development of regional trauma care systems in the United States.

LESSON: Getting the patient to the right health care facility helps
          prevent injury mortality.

7.3. Anesthesia

In the late 1970s and early 1980s record numbers of patients began to sue anesthesiologists for malpractice; as a result, malpractice premiums for anesthesiologists skyrocketed, becoming the most expensive in medicine. In 1982 the ABC television news magazine 20/20 aired a segment highlighting shoddy anesthesia practices at several institutions.

In the mid-1980s the major malpractice carrier for the nine Boston hospitals affiliated with Harvard Medical School helped spur Harvard physicians to create the first set of comprehensive practice standards for the field; these standards quickly gained broad currency. Standardization of existing equipment, better training (e.g., simulators), and new monitoring technology (e.g., pulse oximetry, which uses a small clip on the patient's fingertip to measure oxygen in the blood, and capnography, a companion device, which measures carbon dioxide in the blood) were key in helping to reduce mistakes. The visible commitment of the professional society to rapid and continued reduction in physician error appears to have been crucial for success.

It is estimated that patient death rates have declined from 2 per 10,000 anesthetics administered in the early 1980s to 1 in 200,000 by the late 1990s, a drop of almost 98 percent! Whereas anesthesiologists paid about $30,000 per year for malpractice insurance in the early 1980s, that rate fell to about $5,000 to $10,000 by the late 1990s.

LESSON: Tort law sometimes provides financial incentives
          to effectively reduce injury.

7.4. The Jaipur Foot

In war zones in Afghanistan, Rwanda, and Cambodia losing a foot to a land mine is too common an occurrence. Many people in such areas of conflict may never have heard of Chicago or London, but they are likely to know of a town in northern India named Jaipur. Jaipur is famous as the birthplace of an artificial limb, the Jaipur foot, that has dramatically improved the lives of amputees.

In the 1960s the artificial limbs available to below-the-ankle amputees in India were expensive and did not permit much mobility. The "shoe" attached to the limb was made of heavy sponge, making it worthless for a farmer working in the rain or irrigated paddies. It was also a cultural misfit for Indians who sit, eat, sleep, and worship on the floor, all without wearing shoes.

Dr. Pramod Sethi, a surgeon, and Ram Chandra, a sculptor and craftsman, worked together to create a simple, cheap, and easily made artificial foot. In 1969 they created a rubber foot around a hinged wooden ankle that is lightweight, rugged, mobile, and inexpensive. It is waterproof and abrasion-resistant. The amputee can use the foot almost immediately, with little or no training. Those who wear the foot can run, climb trees, and pedal bicycles.

The limb can be built and fitted to the patient in less than an hour and is durable enough to last for more than five years. It can be made from locally available material (e.g., discarded rubber tires and other industrial debris) and fashioned by any reasonably effective local craftsman. Indeed, Sethi's rehabilitation center trains amputees from street beggars to middle-class housewives on how to make the foot. The Jaipur foot has never been patented, which keeps its cost low.

The Jaipur foot gained worldwide fame when the International Committee of the Red Cross began using it extensively in Afghanistan, and subsequently in other war areas such as Iraq, Kargil, India, and the Middle East. Today the Jaipur foot is a convenient way of naming a whole class of handcrafted prosthetics that evoke the human foot exceptionally well in both form and function and yet are cheaper than a pair of Indian shoes.

The Jaipur foot received more publicity when the celebrated Indian dancer and actor Sudha Chandra got a new lease on life after she was fitted with a Jaipur foot. She performed a difficult dance sequence in the film *Nache Mayuri* thanks to this artificial limb. In 1981 Dr. Sethi won the Ramon Magsaysay Award, considered the "Asian Nobel," for the Jaipur foot, a major advance in rehabilitation medicine and medical technology.

Today more than seventy thousand amputees in India alone, many of them migrant laborers injured from falling off moving trains, wear the Jaipur foot. It is listed in *Guinness World Records* for the number of people around the world using this artificial limb.

In the 1960s Indians who lost a foot became effectively crippled; most could not find work, and many became beggars. Over the past decades the Jaipur foot has substantially improved the lives of hundreds of thousands of landmine and other injury victims in the developing world who could never have afforded a more traditional prosthesis.

LESSON: Rehabilitation can reduce the social as well as the physical problems of injury.

HEROES

7.a. Baron Larrey (1766–1842)

Dominique Jean Larrey was surgeon-in-chief of the Napoleonic armies from 1797 until 1815, helping the wounded during sixty battles and more than four hundred engagements. Larrey initiated the Army Ambulance Corps, field hospitals, and the modern method of army surgery. He is considered the father of modern military medicine.

In earlier times, when swords and arrows created most battlefield injuries, soldiers usually took care of their own wounds. With the advent of gunpowder, wounds were often more serious and more quickly susceptible to infection. Still, in the 1790s military regulations required that military hospitals be at least one league distant from the army, and the wounded were left on the field until after the engagement ended. However, in his first battle, Larrey did not wait until the casualties were brought to him at the rear of the field. Instead, he raced into the field to help the wounded. Although his superiors criticized his behavior, the soldiers expressed their gratitude.

Inspired by the speed with which carriages of the French "flying artillery" maneuvered on the battlefield, as surgeon-in-chief Larrey decided to create a "flying ambulance" corps that could quickly treat and then evacuate the wounded to receive more intensive medical care. This method was revolutionary and saved many wounded soldiers who would previously have suffered for hours or days without receiving any medical attention. And Larrey's radical method for triage was to start treating the most dangerously injured, without regard to rank or distinction. Larrey effectively created the forerunner of modern MASH units.

Larrey willingly took care of all those wounded, whether friend or foe. At the battle of Waterloo he was taken prisoner by the Prussians, who might have executed him. His life was saved by Marshal Blucher; Dr. Larrey had saved the marshal's son on the battlefield a few years earlier.

Many historians credit Larrey for providing the impetus that led to the creation of the International Red Cross (1864) and the Geneva Convention (1949), which requires that all wounded enemy soldiers receive medical care.

Larrey instituted many medical advances. He advocated amputating shattered limbs within the first four hours instead of the customary ten to twenty days. Early amputation was technically easier, less painful, less bloody, and far less dangerous. It converted a mangled mess into a well-ordered wound that was less prone to infection and permitted mobility. Larrey also observed that legs frozen stiff felt almost no pain during amputation, so he packed the stumps in ice and snow to diminish the pain. He was one of the first surgeons to extract bullets from wounds by making a counter-opening instead of probing the torn entry path of the bullet. Larrey also recognized the importance of frequently changing bandages and carefully cleaning wounds. He instituted the separation of wounded patients from those suffering from contagious disease.

Larrey himself was a speedy and effective surgeon. During the catastrophic retreat of the French Army from the Russian front, he is reputed to have performed two hundred amputations in a twenty-four-hour period. He was the first surgeon to succeed in amputating a leg at the hip, and made a multitude of innovations in the treatment of leg fracture. Soldiers gave him the nickname "Savior."

After the battles of Lutzen and Bautzen (1813) many soldiers were accused of self-mutilation in order to avoid the real fighting and were sent to be executed. Larrey single-handedly went against the emperor, the highest military authorities, and their concurring physicians. Armed with his undisputed honesty, professional authority, and exceptional reputation, he was able to show that the men had not hurt themselves but had been wounded in battle, thus saving the lives of many innocent soldiers.

The high morale, and therefore the success, of Napoleon's troops was in an important way dependent on Larrey's superb medical care of the wounded. Napoleon had the greatest regard for Larrey: "Larrey was the most honest man and the best friend to the soldier that I ever knew. . . . He is the worthiest man I ever met" (quoted in Faria 1990, 695). Napoleon made Larrey a baron on the field of Wagram in 1809. Today he is considered to be "the first and probably the greatest military surgeon in history" (Skandalakis et al. 2006, 1398).

7.b. Florence Nightingale (1820–1910)

Florence Nightingale was the daughter of a wealthy and well-connected British landowner. Having no son, he made sure Florence was educated in history, philosophy, and mathematics, as well as in five languages. At age 17, she felt herself called by God to some unknown great cause. She rebelled against the expected role for women of her status, which was to become an obedient wife.

To her parents' chagrin, she not only refused to marry several suitors, but decided to become a nurse. Nurses were generally poor women; army nurses were typically hangers-on who followed the soldiers. These women were likely to also serve as cooks or prostitutes. Nightingale went to Germany and studied to become a nurse and then became an unpaid superintendent of a hospital for ill women in London.

In 1853 Russia invaded Turkey; Britain and France sent troops to Turkey in what became known as the Crimean War. Reports of horrific conditions for the wounded led the British secretary of war to send Nightingale, along with thirty-eight volunteer nurses trained by her, to Turkey. Nightingale found medicines in short supply, lax hygiene, and mass infections.

Doctors and military officers objected to Nightingale's plans for reforming the hospitals. She used her contacts at the London *Times* to report on the way the British Army was treating its wounded soldiers. After much publicity Nightingale was given the task of organizing the hospital. She began by thoroughly cleaning both hospital and equipment. With her own money she set up huge boilers to destroy lice. She believed that by keeping patients well-fed, warm, comfortable, and above all clean, nursing could solve many of the problems that nineteenth-century medicine could not. Such interventions—washing and bathing the soldiers, laundering their linens, feeding them, and giving them a clean bed to lie in—today seem like acts of common sense and common kindness, but were little short of revolutionary at the time.

The main hospital at Scutari was overcrowded and built over sewers with little ventilation. Nightingale attempted to disinfect the floors, but the wooden planks were so rotten it was impossible. A few months after her taking charge of the hospital a sanitary commission made recommendations, such as flushing out the sewers, that Nightingale quickly carried out. She later discovered that the major factor in reducing the hospital death rate was these improvements in hygiene.

Nightingale's work inspired massive public support throughout England. A letter to the *Times* in 1855 on her activities illustrates why: "Wherever there is disease in its most dangerous form, and the hand of the spoiler distressingly nigh, there is that incomparable woman sure to be seen; her benignant presence is an influence for good comfort even amid the struggles of expiring nature. She is a ministering angel without any exaggeration in these hospitals, and as her slender form glides quietly along each corridor, every fellow's face softens with gratitude at the sight of her."

Nightingale returned to Britain in 1857 as a national heroine. That same year, in his poem "Santa Filomena," Henry Wadsworth Longfellow immortalized her as the "Lady with a Lamp": "So in that house of misery/A lady with a lamp I see/Pass through the glimmering gloom/And flit from room to room."

On her return home she wrote the Royal Commission's report that led to a major overhaul of army military care, the establishment of an Army Medical School, and a comprehensive system of army medical records. In 1859 she created what became the Nightingale School of Nursing, and in 1860 her book *Notes on Nursing* was published, which served as a cornerstone of the curriculum for that and subsequent nursing schools.

Nightingale is remembered for her compassion and care, along with strong administrative skills. One of her major contributions to the world was her role in founding the modern nursing profession. She set a shining example for nurses everywhere of compassion, commitment to patient care, and diligent and thoughtful hospital administration.

Nightingale had a gift for mathematics and statistics. She was a pioneer in the visual presentation of information, popularizing the polar area chart (similar to today's pie chart) to depict patient outcome changes caused by the improvements in hospital care. She helped popularize the idea that social phenomena could be objectively measured and subject to mathematical analysis. Later in her life she made a comprehensive statistical study of sanitation in rural India and was the leading figure in the introduction of improved medical care and public health service there.

Nightingale's two greatest life accomplishments, reforming hospitals and pioneering modern nursing, were notable given that most Victorian women did not attend college or pursue professional careers. Her career inspired many others. Henri Dunant, founder of the Red Cross and the originator of the Geneva Convention, said in 1864, "I feel emboldened to pay my homage. To Miss Nightingale I give all the honor of this humane Convention. It was her work in the Crimea that inspired me."

In 1915 Mohandas K. Gandhi wrote this about Florence Nightingale:

> Born of a noble and rich family, she gave up her life of ease and comfort and set out to nurse the wounded and ailing. . . . She rendered strenuous service in the Battle of Inkerman. At that time there were neither beds nor other amenities for the wounded. There were 10,000 wounded under the

charge of this single woman. . . . If bleeding could be stopped, the wounds bandaged and the requisite diet given, the lives of many thousands would doubtless be saved. The only thing necessary was kindness and nursing, which Miss Nightingale provided. . . . No wonder that a country where such women are born is prosperous. (Dossey 1999, 415)

7.c. Peter Safar (1924–2003)

Anesthesiologist Peter Safar was a pioneer in developing systems of pre-hospital and hospital care, in particular cardiopulmonary resuscitation (CPR), ambulance service, and intensive care units (ICUs).

Cardiopulmonary Resuscitation   Early in his career Safar learned "that the anesthesiology used in the operating room can be applied effectively outside the operating room. That led to an interest in resuscitation" (Mitka 2003, 2485). His interest in resuscitation outside the hospital led him to seek methods that could be taught to laypersons to bring resuscitation medicine into the streets in the form of life-supporting first aid. Safar wanted the public to be able to assist and intervene when someone suffered trauma. First he had to determine what they should do.

In 1956 Safar began human experiments to determine which methods of resuscitation would work best. In an approach that would not be allowed today, seated volunteers were given curare to paralyze the breathing muscles, while the heart continued to beat. Safar compared the accepted arm-lift method with mouth-to-mouth ventilation. His article, published in the *Journal of the American Medical Association* in 1958, helped convince the world of the best approach to resuscitation.

Modern CPR consists of three steps: the ABCs of airway, breathing, and circulation. Safar's research formed the basis for the first two steps: the head tilt and chin lift to open an obstructed airway (Step A), and mouth-to-mouth breathing as a form of artificial respiration (Step B). From behind the Iron Curtain the Russian resuscitation expert Vladimir Negovsky tested the third step: artificial circulation (Step C). This third step consists of chest compressions, pushing down on the sternum with two hands, in an attempt to circulate oxygenated blood to the vital organs in the body. The work of Negovsky and Safar was nominated three times for the Nobel Prize in Medicine.

Safar is credited with putting the three steps together. He not only demonstrated that CPR worked, but he successfully pushed for its widespread use. In 1957 he wrote the book *ABC of Resuscitation*, which established the basis for mass training of CPR techniques. He is often called the father of CPR.

Safar influenced a Norwegian toy maker, Asmund Laerdal, to develop a realistic mannequin for CPR training. Many students have been taught to determine if a patient is unconscious by gently shaking this Resusci-Anne doll and calling, "Annie, Annie, are you OK?"

Ambulance Service   In the late 1950s the ill and injured throughout the United States were being transported to hospitals in station wagons or even hearses, with no treatment given en route. Working with the Baltimore Fire Department ambulance service, Safar helped design a modern ambulance, with a large compartment for a bed and seating for the attendant. It had an oxygen source and equipment to insert an airway tube to support breathing. The attendants were taught intubation and basic CPR.

In the 1970s Safar was responsible for establishing the first ambulance service manned by trained attendants in the city of Pittsburgh. He trained so-called unemployable black recruits from Pittsburgh's impoverished inner city. With a federal grant he empowered these poor, young minority men with the skills and confidence to succeed. "Despite tremendous political pressure against him coming from the highest levels of the white establishment in Pittsburgh, who wanted to see the 'Freedom House Ambulance Service' fail, it proved a resounding success" (Pretto 2005, 83).

ICUs   Prior to 1958 the postanesthesia recovery room was not staffed at night; that year Safar established what is considered the first intensive care unit in the United States, in Baltimore. It was physician-staffed around the clock for the prolonged care of patients with life-threatening injuries and illnesses. Soon ICUs were instituted in Boston, Toronto, Auckland, New Zealand, and elsewhere.

Safar was a giant in many diverse areas, and much beloved by his colleagues. They created some two dozen catch phrases that captured Safar's philosophy of life. Dubbed "Peter's Laws for the Navigation of Life," Law 15 stated, "Bureaucracy is a challenge to be conquered with a righteous attitude, a tolerance for stupidity, and a bulldozer when necessary." Law 22 was: "It's up to us to save the world."

7.d. Jeffrey Cooper (1946–) and Ellison C. (Jeep) Pierce Jr. (1928–)

Over the past two decades, the large gains in safety for patients under anesthesia are due to the collective effort of the anesthesiology community.

But two individuals who deserve special recognition are Jeffrey Cooper and Ellison C. Pierce Jr.

Jeffrey Cooper is an engineer who in 1978 was the lead author of a seminal article entitled "Preventable Anesthesia Mishaps: A Study of Human Factors." His detailed analysis of over 350 mistakes was the first in-depth scientific analysis of errors in medicine. Contrary to conventional wisdom, Cooper found that most problems did not occur when the anesthetic is first administered ("takeoff"), but in the middle stages of narcosis, when the anesthetist's attention starts to fade. Some of the worst errors were in ventilation, often the result of incorrectly connected or leaky breathing tubes. Cooper documented that many of the anesthesia machines were not standardized and poorly designed; for example, in about half the machines a clockwise turn increased the concentration of anesthetic, while in the others a clockwise turn decreased the concentration.

Although Cooper's study provoked widespread discussion there was no concerted effort to solve the various problems he had exposed until Dr. Ellison (Jeep) Pierce Jr. was elected vice president of the American Society of Anesthesiologists (ASA). Since beginning his practice in 1960, Pierce had maintained a case file on details from all the deadly anesthetic accidents he had come across. One case was particularly troublesome: friends had taken their 18-year-old daughter to the hospital to have her wisdom teeth pulled under general anesthesia. The anesthesiologist inserted the breathing tube into her esophagus instead of her trachea, which sometimes occurs. But tragically, and far more rarely, the anesthesiologist failed to recognize and correct the error. Deprived of oxygen, the girl died within minutes.

As ASA vice president, Pierce budgeted funds to solve the problems identified by Cooper. An international conference gathered ideas from around the world, and anesthesia machine designers were brought into the discussion. Many changes were instituted, making it less likely for anesthesiologists to make errors and more likely for them to detect any errors that were made. Dials on machines were standardized; locks prevented accidental administration of more than one gas; controls prevented oxygen delivery to be turned down to zero; and monitors were provided that tracked blood oxygen levels to provide early warning signs of problems with the patient's breathing.

Pierce helped institutionalize the patient safety movement. He set an important precedent in anesthesiology by creating the Committee on Patient Safety and Risk Management, the first such committee of its kind in any health care organization, and the Anesthesia Patient Safety Foundation

(APSF). Under his direction, the APSF deserves much of the credit for promoting oximetry and other monitoring devices in the operating room.

In his acceptance speech for the Public Interest in Anesthesia Award, Cooper emphasized the importance of *institutionalizing* a "systems approach" to patient safety: "All of us who work in patient safety must understand that safety is a never ending effort. . . . We must be ever vigilant to identify the system issues that undermine safety. We must work to create organizations and cultures that have as their first priority the safety of all patients" ("Cooper Receives" 2003).

7.e. Lucian Leape (1930–)

One of the many people who have made a difference in public health is Dr. Lucian Leape. Leape entered pediatric surgery when it was just becoming a specialty. Too many times he found himself rebuilding an esophagus for a toddler who had swallowed liquid lye drain cleaner. Making his first foray into the field of public health, Leape went to the laboratory and found that lye kills esophageal cells within seconds; discovering an antidote was not going to be the answer to this problem. The effective way to prevent these injuries was to change the product or get rid of it altogether. In a 1971 article in the *New England Journal of Medicine* he quantified the number of victims, the circumstances of ingestion, and the extent of the devastating, irreversible injuries to these children (Leape et al. 1971). With the help of Senator Robert Dole Leape was able to persuade the U.S. Consumer Product Commission to remove the most dangerous forms of concentrated liquid lye from the retail market. Although hundreds of children were saved, the manufacturers "went after me to prove I had a bad character" (quoted in Herman 2000, 25).

In the 1980s, after two decades in surgery, Leape decided to leave his clinical practice and focus on broader issues of medical practice. He has become "generally known as the father of the modern patient safety movement" (Wachter 2007). A main goal of this movement is to reduce medical error by improving the systems of organization in hospitals and other medical settings. Leape believes that it is not just particular methods that need to be changed, but an entrenched medical culture.

Leape worked on a landmark medical practice study that examined thirty thousand patient records. Some 4 percent of the patients had adverse events, and 66 percent of these were caused by medical error. His article in the *Journal of the American Medical Association* (Leape 1994) promoted the human factors approach, also called the injury prevention approach, that begins with the premise that human errors are inevitable. But instead of blaming the physician, Leape advised creating a system in which it is difficult rather than easy for physicians to make errors and in which errors do not lead to serious injury.

This focus on physician error was controversial in medicine. Hospitals and physicians were resistant to admitting mistakes and making the needed changes. Indeed, the culture was that physicians weren't supposed to make errors, and if they did, it wasn't to be talked about. Leape was told not to use the word "error' in his *JAMA* article, but that was what the article was about. "It's not pleasant to be ostracized by your colleagues. He went out on a limb. Here's a guy who's changing the world" (Berwick, cited in Herman 2000, 30).

Leape has recently written about health care providers' accountability and the importance of apologizing to patients for errors. He sees the need for a systems approach even when focusing on individual accountability. "We do not have good systems for making sure [doctors] are well trained and maintain competency. We don't have good systems for assessing their performance. We don't have good systems for helping them." The key is still to get beyond the notions of blame and punishment.

Leape was an advisor for the Hundred Thousand Lives Campaign organized by the Institute for Healthcare Improvement, headed by Don Berwick. This nationwide initiative launched in 2004 encouraged hospitals to implement various best practices to prevent adverse drug events, surgical site infections, central line infections, ventilator-associated pneumonia, and other problems to reduce patient morbidity and mortality. The success of that initiative led in late 2006 to the even more ambitious 5 Million Lives Campaign to improve hospital care to reduce surgical complications and reduce harm from high-alert medications and other problems in order to protect patients from millions of incidents of medical harm.

In 2003 Leape received the DuPont Award for Excellence in Children's Health Care. The following year he received the John Eisenberg Patient Safety Award and *Modern Healthcare* named him one of the one hundred most powerful people in health care.

7.f. Subroto Das (1965–)

In the past few decades in India a rapid increase in the number of motor vehicles and a large expansion in the road network have led to a steep rise in road crashes. Currently some eighty-five thousand individuals are killed annually in motor vehicle collisions.

Fatalities could be reduced by a variety of measures, including compulsory seat belt laws, a reduction in drinking and driving, and safer vehicle design. Pedestrians could be protected with separate paths and lanes, and injured people could be saved with improvements in the medical care system. In India only 20 percent of traffic fatalities are killed outright; most lives are lost because victims do not receive adequate medical care during the "golden hour" after the initial injury.

Dr. Subroto Das, a physician with training in hospital administration, lost a friend in a road accident when medical help did not arrive in time. Then in 1999 he and his wife, Sushmita, were involved in a traffic collision. They lay injured by the side of a busy road for four hours before a kindly milkman stopped to help. Even after that it took hours before they reached a hospital. They decided they could not let such misfortune befall others.

India lacks a standardized emergency response system; for example, there is no central call line such as 911, and there are no clear rules as to who is responsible for the evacuation of accident victims. An emergency medical system (EMS) barely exists in much of the country, and when it does function, the red tape of bureaucracy often makes it ineffective. For example, an ambulance may take a critically injured victim to a hospital two hours away rather than to one ten minutes away in a neighboring state. Most ambulances lack both trained personnel and good medical equipment.

Das and his wife are working to build a comprehensive system of emergency care through the Highway Rescue Project. The goal is to eliminate any obstacle that stands in the way of rapid response to postaccident trauma. Das has helped organize police, firefighters, and ambulance owners and drivers to ensure that they can save lives without falling into jurisdictional disputes. He has mapped the highways, set up a twenty-four-hour telephone help line, and worked to ensure the adequacy of every hospital, clinic, and blood bank near the highways. He has even trained schoolchildren in the villages along the highways in primary first aid, making methods of saving lives an integral part of their education.

Beginning in 2002 the program was successfully implemented along a 1,300-kilometer stretch of national highways, with plans to widen it to 15,000 kilometers. In its first three years the program helped over a thousand accident victims with life-threatening injuries. Das received India's 2004 International Road Safety Award.

CHAPTER 8

Models of Injury Prevention

INTRODUCTION

This chapter describes five injury prevention initiatives that have served as models for others. The five are an industry success: airlines; a town success: Harstad, Norway; a city success: Boston; and two country successes: Sweden and the Netherlands. Four of the five successes concern unintentional injuries; the Boston success deals with youth gun violence prevention.

The airline success has served as an example for medicine, which is trying to reduce provider error and increase safety. Boston's successful approach to firearm violence prevention was rolled out to other cities. Other jurisdictions have attempted to emulate the Scandinavian successes.

Most of the other successes in this book deal with single initiatives (e.g., bike helmets, child safety caps, energy-absorbing steering columns, minimum legal drinking age). The five models in this chapter describe a broader systems approach. While most of the other chapters deal with tactics (single policies), this chapter deals with strategy (multiple initiatives). Other successes in this book with a broad strategic element include 3.3 Building the Golden Gate Bridge; 4.9 Child Injuries in Harlem; 6.1 Suicide in the Air Force; 6.5 Nightclub Violence, and 7.3 Anesthesia.

The successes in this chapter show the importance of gathering good data consistently over time, having committed leadership, and inducing all the stakeholders to cooperate. They demonstrate that incredible accomplishments are possible when safety becomes a top priority and people actively join together to prevent injuries and violence.

BLUEPRINTS FOR SUCCESS

8.1. Industry: Airlines

On January 13, 1982, a flight from Washington, DC, to Fort Lauderdale, Florida, crashed into the 14th Street Bridge, which connects the District of Colombia and Arlington, Virginia, and plunged into the ice-covered Potomac River. The National Transportation Safety Board (NTSB) determined that the probable cause of the accident was the flight crew's failure to use engine anti-ice, their decision to take off with ice on the aircraft, and the captain's failure to abort the takeoff when his attention was called to anomalous engine instrument readings. Contributing to the accident were the prolonged ground delay, the pitch-up characteristics of the B-737 aircraft when the leading edge has even small amounts of snow or ice, and the limited experience of the flight crew in winter operations.

Airline safety is heavily regulated in the United States. The Federal Aviation Administration (FAA), with a budget of some $14 billion in FY 2008, is responsible for the safety of civil aviation. The NTSB investigates every civil aviation accident in the United States and issues recommendations to the FAA. It has the federal mandate and subpoena power to investigate and make public the probable cause of all crashes.

The airline industry has large economic incentives to improve safety. Air crashes are newsworthy. Airlines and aircraft manufacturers lose customers when their safety comes into question, and insurance companies often raise premiums. Airline stock prices fall after major catastrophes. Even absent FAA inspections and fines, airline executives ignore safety at their own peril (Mitchell & Maloney 1989; Hemenway 1993).

Airline safety in the United States has improved over the past eighty years due to a wide variety of factors: planes are safer, runways are better, and radar and other navigational equipment have improved over time. The airline approach to safety has become a model for other industries, such as medicine (Institute of Medicine 2000). A few of the many interrelated aspects of the airline safety model are highlighted below:

1. Every accident receives an in-depth investigation by an independent authority. Much information can be gleaned by in-depth investigations into each rare but tragic plane crash. Before 1940 the FAA performed such investigations, but often kept the reports secret so as not to damage the public image of aviation and to prevent the information getting into the hands of attorneys representing victims suing the airlines. In 1974 the

NTSB became a fully independent agency, completely separate from the FAA and the Department of Transportation. It is thus better able to perform objective evaluations, establish probable cause free of political interference, and make its findings available to the public. It has no power to punish, or to assign legal or moral responsibility, or to force the FAA to implement any of its recommendations.

2. Mistakes and near-misses are also carefully analyzed. Shortly after becoming a fully independent agency, the NTSB proposed the creation of a database of close calls and other dangerous events. Analysis of this information permits the dissemination of solutions to problems before they became actual accidents. Each near-miss now demands explanation and action. As an independent agency, the NTSB has no stake in trying to cover up near-miss incidents or actual accidents (Lacey 2007).

3. The data system includes most near-misses because of blame-free reporting. Historically the FAA urged pilots to report any close call (to help identify threats to safety), while simultaneously subjecting them to prosecution for regulatory violations based on their own self-reports. To overcome the reluctance of pilots to hurt themselves and their airlines by reporting near-misses, the Aviation Safety Reporting System (ASRS), a confidential, nonpunitive reporting system, was created. It is voluntary, although it is promoted as a professional obligation (e.g., in pilot training), and pilots are given limited immunity from FAA prosecution. Specific pilots and airlines are not identified in the reports. The objective of ASRS is to promote learning from experience rather than to discipline individuals for regulatory infractions (Tamuz 2007).

4. Expert observers often ride along in the cockpit. An additional source of data comes from observations of activity during normal flights. These confidential data confirm that danger, and error, are common, averaging about two per flight. The types of errors discovered include the pilot's entering the wrong information in the flight computer, misunderstanding altitude clearance, and not avoiding bad weather. Identifying and helping to correct such errors are critical to preventing accidents (Helmreich 2000).

5. Airline personnel are trained in teamwork. In the late 1970s it became clear that most airline disasters resulted not from

mechanical failure or the pilot's lack of technical skill, but from errors associated with breakdowns in communication, decision making, and leadership. It can be said that it is the team, not the aircraft or the individual pilot, that is at the root of most accidents. Historically pilot training dealt with only the technical aspects of flying. Now training includes a focus on countermeasures to error, such as cross-checking, monitoring, briefings (in which the person in charge reviews the tasks facing the team and highlights the potential threats), and interpersonal communication methods. The training also includes methods to improve the work group culture. Commercial airline pilots are taught, among other things, to recognize the impact of fatigue, to effectively communicate problems, to resolve conflicts, to develop contingency plans, and to listen to team members. Subordinates are taught how to raise safety concerns and how to question the actions of authority figures without challenging their authority.

6. Pilots are trained with sophisticated simulators. These simulators allow crews to practice dealing with error-inducing situations and to receive feedback on both their individual and team performance. The simulators provide experience for real-life stress situations without the real-life danger of crashing the plane.

7. The airlines' approach to safety is a systems approach. Accidents rarely result from a single failure or action; they result from a combination of things, for example, an error in maintenance that causes a failure in flight that a member of the flight crew then responds to incorrectly. Accidents result from a chain of events that provide multiple opportunities for prevention. Remove any link in the chain and the accident is avoided. The airlines try to remove all the links.

The yearly average number of fatalities per billion miles on passenger and cargo airlines has fallen dramatically each decade (Table 4), totaling over 99.9 percent in eight decades—an incredible success story. Air transport is now far safer than travel by automobile. Per mile, you are about twenty-four times more likely to die traveling by automobile than by commercial airline (Borowsky & Gaynor 2007).

However, the aviation safety system is still far from ideal. On the NTSB website, for example, is a list of Most Wanted Transportation Safety Improvements. In the aviation area, as of April 2007, these

TABLE 4

U.S. airline fatalities

Average yearly fatalities per billion aircraft miles	
1927–1929	920
1930s	170
1940s	26
1950s	9.5
1960s	5.6
1970s	1.8
1980s	0.9
1990s	0.6
2000–2006	0.2

NOTE: Passenger and cargo airlines operating under 14 CFR 121. Excludes illegal acts such as suicide, sabotage, and terrorism. In 2006 these planes flew 8 billion miles, the equivalent of 2.6 million trips across the continental U.S.
SOURCE: "Safety Record" 2007.

included specific methods to reduce the dangers to aircraft flying in icing conditions, to stop runway incursions, and to reduce accidents caused by human fatigue. These are currently listed as having an unacceptable response from the FAA; that is, the NTSB believes the FAA hasn't done enough to help the airlines correct these problems.

LESSON: A systems approach with lots of good policies and good incentives can lead to a dramatic improvement in safety.

8.2. Town: Harstad, Norway

In 1985 Harstad, a small Norwegian town (22,000 inhabitants) 150 miles north of the Artic Circle, initiated a community-based injury prevention program. A local group was established with representatives from the area hospital as well as public and private organizations (e.g., insurance companies) and interested individuals. The group actively used injury data to guide and evaluate their efforts. Three of the major injury areas they decided to focus on were burns to small children, falls and fractures in the elderly, and traffic injuries.

Burns   The group gathered medical information on the extent of the problem as well as the exact circumstances of the scalds and burns (e.g., "The toddler pulled down the coffee kettle from the stove and was scalded"). Key to the campaign were public health nurses, who vaccinate virtually all Norwegian children and visit the home every four months for the first four years of a child's life. The nurses provided extensive counseling on the circumstances of child burns in the community. Examples of practical advice included avoiding drinking hot beverages with a child on the lap and setting the table for tea or coffee without a tablecloth. Two specific passive interventions were promoted: the purchase and installation of guard rails around the edge of the stove and lowering the temperature of the tap water thermostat. The nurses went to electrical appliance stores to ensure the availability of the cooker safeguards.

Program messages were also conveyed face to face in shopping malls, at health fairs, and in doctors' offices. Press releases by the group on the progress of the intervention were highlighted in the local media.

The child injury burn rate to Harstad children fell over 50 percent compared with a slight increase in the control community that had not intervened to reduce child burns. Rates of burn injury in Harstad fell most for the more severe stove and tap water scalds.

Falls and Fractures   Health personnel in Harstad were trained in fall and fracture prevention and in 1991 over 80 percent of Harstad residents ages 75–79 accepted the offer of a home visit by these nurses and other trained personnel. More than 750 high-risk elderly people received multiple visits. The aim of the visits was to promote environmental safety, a healthy diet and lifestyle, and a reduction in inactivity and isolation. Safety items, such as anti-slide material on floors and grab bars for stairs and bathrooms were made available. Retirees who were skilled in manual work were also available at one-third of the market price to make recommended physical improvements. Safety boots with spiked soles designed for walking on icy pavements were actively promoted. In addition, a special health station was established for Harstad senior citizens for routine health consultations, and physiotherapists offered weekly workout sessions in gymnasia.

Many voluntary organizations, including church groups, the pensioners' society, and the Lions Club, actively promoted these efforts. Fracture rates among the elderly in private homes fell 26 percent. Elderly fractures in the control community increased during the period.

Traffic Safety   A variety of traffic safety initiatives were undertaken. One component was education; for example, a popular rally driver, people with paraplegia, police, and surgeons provided information to young drivers at a large city event and in secondary schools. The local motorcycle club promoted helmet use and their safety activities were lauded in the local newspaper. Probably most important, a quarterly *Traffic Injury Report* with detailed information about every hospital-treated traffic injury in the city was sent to every household every season of the year. Local pressure groups used the geographical data to justify demands for a safer physical environment, particularly for children.

Local planners and the police helped make traffic safer. For example, there were increased restrictions on beer sales in grocery stores and curfews for serving alcohol in bars. Separate pedestrian and cyclist roads were built, road bumps were installed, speed limits were lowered, and speed limit enforcement was increased. Conspicuous warning signs were placed on particularly dangerous road segments. After the intervention Harstad residents had higher awareness of and positive attitudes toward safety issues (e.g., drinking alcohol and driving, speeding) compared with residents in the control city. Most important, over the ten-year period traffic injury rates to Harstad children fell 59 percent; overall rates for all ages fell 37 percent. Rates in the control city were largely unchanged.

LESSON: It is possible for a community to effectively mobilize to increase the safety and well-being of its children, its elderly, indeed its entire population.

8.3. City: Boston and Youth Homicide

Like many American cities, Boston saw a large increase in youth homicide in the late 1980s and early 1990s, particularly in poor and minority neighborhoods. The epidemic of youth homicide was probably initiated in the mid-1980s by the arrival of crack cocaine, but the epidemic was maintained by the presence of gangs, guns, and fear.

The initial police response—stopping and searching groups of minority youth for firearms—fueled racial tensions and did little to reduce the deadly violence. Community members were angry and frustrated as gangs increasingly controlled the streets and the police seemed both racist and ineffective.

In the early 1990s more adults began working in the streets of Boston to help reduce the violence. The mayor created a group called Boston Street Workers, mostly young men not too far removed from gang life themselves, whose job it was to connect with and help at-risk youth. Police increased their community policing, and probation officers began spending more time on the streets at night. After a shooting at a church it became clear that the church needed to take its message to the street, or else the street would bring its message into the church. Black clergy formed the Ten Point Coalition and began walking the streets at night. These groups of adults—police, probation, Street Workers, and clergy— often at odds in the past, were all out on the street when there were shootings. They learned to talk to and respect each other.

Most important, they began forming alliances. Probation officers, formerly seen as fuzzy headed 9–5 social worker types by the police, began riding in squad cars, working with the police to enforce the terms of probation. And police went with the probation officers to the homes of the youth and began to see these gang members as struggling kids, not just criminals.

The Street Workers and the clergy worked together. The street workers had connections to the kids who needed resources, and the churches had the resources and the desire to reach the same kids. The clergy, for example, provided vans and tickets for events because, as one Street Worker put it, "Even though these kids are carrying guns and selling drugs, they're nothing but kids. You have to give them an opportunity to be a kid again, to see what a kid's life is like. And we didn't have that from anybody but the ministers" (Pruitt 2001, 14).

Given the stormy history of the Boston police and the black community, perhaps the most significant alliance was that between police and the Ten Point Coalition. Where previously these clergy had organized public hearings on charges of police misconduct, the Ten Point Coalition instituted an awards ceremony for exemplary police and youth leaders. The Ten Point Coalition also began to acknowledge publicly that some of the young men in gangs simply could not be saved on the street: they had to be arrested and removed from the community.

Police attitudes were also changing. In 1994 the new police commissioner visited the areas with the most violence and asked the police there what they needed. Fully expecting to hear "more cops, more tough judges," he was astonished to hear these hardened gang cops say "We need jobs and alternatives for these kids" (Pruitt 2001, 16). Over time police work in Boston's inner city began to be as much about prevention as about law enforcement. The shift in emphasis found licensed social workers in precinct stations and made the Boston Police Department a leading player in finding jobs for kids at risk.

Probably the tipping point in the struggle to reduce lethal youth violence in Boston was a problem-oriented policing intervention named Operation Ceasefire. Academic researchers working with a task force composed of key Boston policy makers showed that over 60 percent of youth homicide was gang-related. Yet only about thirteen hundred youth (less than 1 percent of their age group citywide) were gang members. Boston's sixty gangs were small and their members, who were well known to the police, probation officers, and Street Workers, tended to have extensive criminal records. These young men were generally both the perpetrators and the victims of Boston youth homicides; chronic disputes (back-and-forth vendettas or "beefs") among the gangs were the main driver of the lethal violence.

Evidence also pointed to the key role of illicit markets that supplied these youth with firearms and the role of fear in driving these youth to acquire guns for self-defense. Guns among these kids led to many seemingly senseless shootings. "These kids are armed, edgy and believe that they cannot be insulted or walk away from a fight without irretrievably losing face and thereby risking additional victimization" (Kennedy et al. 1996, 154). Although only a tenth or so of gang members were consistently dangerous and frightening, they tended to set the tone for the street life of other gang members and had a dire effect on the community as a whole.

Operation Ceasefire had two main components. One was a focused attack on illegal gun trafficking in Boston, designed to disrupt the market supply of firearms for these youth. Gun traces showed that only about one-third of the crime guns came from Massachusetts; another third from southern states and most of the rest from New England states with permissive firearm laws. Many of the guns used were relatively new. As police routinely tried to obtain information about the chain of distribution of drugs when drug dealers were arrested, they began eliciting information on the chain of distribution of illicit firearms from arrestees. Gun buybacks and amnesties also helped get some of the weapons off the street. Anonymous studies in Boston high schools during this period found that even among youth who admitted illegally carrying guns, the majority wanted to live in a world where it was impossible for them to obtain firearms (Hemenway et al. 1996). This was not currently the world in which they lived.

The second component of the strategy was to send a clear message to all gang members that violence, especially involving firearms, would be severely punished and refraining from violence would be rewarded. The key was to make such a deterrence strategy credible.

While regular police work would continue throughout the city, any gang that brought attention to itself by engaging in serious violence would receive special and unwelcome treatment. Gang members usually had criminal records and were thus very vulnerable to increased legal scrutiny. Crackdowns included probation curfew checks, serving outstanding warrants, street drug law enforcement, and attention to minor violations such as driving an unregistered car or drinking in public. All parts of the criminal justice system acted together to increase arrests and expedite prosecutions for the specific gangs engaging in serious violence. The goal was not to eliminate gangs or stop all gang offending, but to control and deter serious violence.

The strategy involved face-to-face meetings with gangs. It was made quite clear that regular police work would continue throughout the city, but a special gang unit would focus on particular gangs. Although the police could not stop all illegal gang activity, serious gang violence would be the chief determinant of where police would target this resource. Gangs were told, in effect, "We know who you are, we know what you are doing, we can't stop all your offending, but serious violence will no longer be tolerated. We are doing this to protect you. Go and tell your friends." When one gang that had been explicitly warned continued the serious violence, twenty-three members of the gang were arrested on federal and state drug charges. The case was in the paper for weeks, and members of all gangs were sent special flyers so that they would get the message. In another case of serious gang violence the gang leader was arrested for possession of a single bullet and sentenced to twenty years in federal prison with no possibility of parole. This case was also highly publicized.

The approach turned one law enforcement concept on its head. As an assistant to the U.S. attorney for Massachusetts noted, "Normally we think our power is in knowing what we're going to do and not telling anybody, and making sure they, the defendants, don't know what we are doing. This was a very different notion that was based on the premise that people can change, and that people make decisions based on the consequences, if they understand them" (Pruitt 2001, 24). And the message was clear: stop the shooting and the police will stop arresting you for minor infractions.

Key to the success of Operation Ceasefire was that community stakeholders were brought into the deliberations from the beginning, they had important input, and they bought into the final strategy. They were present at the meetings with the gangs and supported the police efforts.

Most important, the youth were offered positive alternatives to a life of violence on the streets. The business community helped with jobs, job training, mentoring, and afterschool programs. Gang members were thus given a clear choice: Stop the serious violence or you will most certainly go to prison; make the right choice and we will help you move away from life on the streets. As one former gang member put it, "I had to choose between my [gang] friends or my future, and I chose my future" (quoted in Pruitt 2001, 26).

A principal concept behind Operation Ceasefire was that gang members were young people in trouble: they did not want to die, and they needed help from adults. One of the programs offered was helping these young men to be good fathers. As one probation officer observed, "Some of these are tough, tough guys. And to have 18 guys sit around and talk about their children, and how they want to be a proud example for their children, and how they want to take responsibility, and how much they want to learn about doing that—it's absolutely eye opening. And it's rejuvenating for somebody like me who's been around for 28 years. It gives me new hope that things can change."

Following Operation Ceasefire youth homicide victimization in Boston fell over 60 percent and remained low for the next eight years. Similar declines were seen in youth gun assaults. The core idea of Operation Ceasefire—that the violence had become a self-sustaining cycle that could be broken—appeared justified. The "Boston Miracle" was hailed nationally as an unprecedented success.

Many people and institutions were important in this success, including the Boston mayors who promoted community policing and supported the Street Workers program, the Boston police chiefs who were willing to innovate, the Boston clergy who worked on the streets, the Roman Catholic cardinal who publicly supported the efforts of the black Protestant clergy in a city with an overwhelmingly Irish Catholic police department, the Boston businesses who provided funds for training and opportunities for employment, the academics who served as research partners, and the Boston grassroots community organizations that worked with troubled youth and taught dispute resolution skills that helped change adolescent norms concerning violence.

As one Street Worker put it, "You can go into those communities now and see grandmothers walking the streets and in the parks that the gangs controlled. I can see six year olds playing again, people out on the streets, in their backyards, having cook-outs, whereas before they were nervous about a stray bullet hitting them or their family" (quoted in Pruitt 2001, 26). Adults who were once too intimated to leave their home became a beneficial street presence in the lives of the youth.

Unfortunately the Boston Miracle lasted for less than a decade. Most of its organizers and major players were promoted or drifted to other jobs or causes; some of its tactics were abandoned, and fiscal limitations cut many key programs. The Street Workers program epitomizes some of the problems; its funding was cut, and the number of workers fell from forty to twelve by 2003. The state mandated that anyone working with children had to have a clean criminal record and the city required Street Workers to have two years of experience working with at-risk youth. These mandates precluded recent former gang members, often the most effective Street Workers, from joining the ranks. The Street Workers joined a union whose rules basically precluded them from working past 9 P.M. By 2005 it was clear that government needed to increase funding, relax the criminal background requirements, and change workers' shifts. Boston homicides, which numbered 152 in 1990, had fallen to 31 in 1999, but by 2005 the number had risen again to 75.

> LESSON: No one organization can solve the problem of youth
>   violence, but a strong commitment along with institutional
>   collaboration—where people leave their stereotypes, as
>   well as their personal and professional egos, at the door—
>   can make the streets a much safer place.

8.4. Country: Sweden

In the 1950s Sweden had higher rates of injury deaths to children ages 1 to 14 than the United States. By the early 1990s the Swedish injury death rate for children had fallen so much that it was 37 percent of the U.S. rate; in other words, an American child was 2.7 times more likely to die due to an injury than a Swedish child. Sweden now has the lowest rate of child injury mortality in the world ("A League Table" 2001; Jansson et al. 2006).

Sweden's remarkable injury success has been ascribed to the systematic safety campaign initiated by the Children's Accident Committee, established in 1954. Their main message was that injury is a public health problem that society as a whole must control.

The goal was to engage existing groups to make child safety their top priority. For example, the Red Cross and the Life Savings Association assumed responsibility for water safety; police, automobile associations, and traffic safety groups took leadership in the traffic safety area. The Swedish government initially provided only minimal support, consistent with the Swedish tradition that new programs are created and tested in the voluntary sector and assumed by government only if they are shown to work.

There were three main aspects of the safety campaign. The first was to create a comprehensive surveillance (data) system of fatal and nonfatal injuries. Data and evaluations of new programs were crucial in gaining support for prevention from politicians, the media, and the public. The second aspect was to use regulation and legislation to make a safer environment for children. Children's protection had to become a major societal goal when roads were built and products designed. The safety campaign emphasized separating children from danger, such as from guns or cars. In many communities, for example, distinct walking and biking paths were built so that children could go from home to school or playground without ever crossing a street. To ensure that products are safe, the Swedish Board of Consumer Policies now tests all household products. The third aspect was to create a broad-based education campaign for the general public, emphasizing the preventability of almost all injuries. Safety messages were stressed by physicians and nurses, as well as by Swedish television, which is filled with self-improvement advice. Since 1991 Sweden has banned TV and radio ads targeted to children.

A developmental approach was undertaken, with persistent education to parents on the need for vigilance over children, whose capricious actions are considered a normal part of growing up. For example, in the 1970s almost every Swedish municipality built a public indoor facility to provide swimming lessons free of charge, and almost all now have outdoor heated facilities. To prevent drowning, all elementary school children were taught to swim, life jackets were promoted and made available at little or no cost, and the need for parents to constantly supervise their children was stressed. Between 1954 and 1988, the child drowning rate in Sweden fell 90 percent; during the same period, the U.S. child drowning rate fell only 5 percent.

In Sweden the safety of children remains a national priority. New homes must incorporate a detailed list of child safety measures, including childproof electrical sockets. Traffic guards ensure the safety of children when they must cross traffic. Publicly organized day care focuses on preventing accidents to children; the percentage of children ages 1 to 7 in registered day care rose from 10 percent in 1965 to 72 percent by the late 1990s. Physical punishment is forbidden in school and at home; the percentage of the Swedish population in favor of physical punishment of children decreased from 53 percent in 1965 to 11 percent in 1994 (Jansson et al. 2006). These and many other initiatives were designed to protect children, and they have succeeded. In 1954 some 450 Swedish children under age 15 died of injuries; by 2000 the number of child injury deaths had fallen to 49 ("Sweden: Progress" 2006).

Because Sweden is a consensus democracy any attempt to steamroll the minority is viewed with distaste. Citizens have respect for rules and social norms. For example, there is no toleration for drinking and driving; both severe governmental penalties and social disapprobation keep alcohol-related traffic injuries low.

Although many Americans view Sweden as a welfare state with socialist leanings, the government actually does not do many things that it might. It provides little money for injury prevention *research;* instead, support for the child safety initiative came from two main sources: automobile manufacturers and insurance companies. In particular, Volvo and Folksam, the insurance company owned largely by Swedish labor unions, provided most of the funding for the initiative. Swedish companies are generally more public-spirited than their American counterparts.

This is also true at the individual level. Compared to Americans, who prize the motto "Every man for himself," the Swedes seem to have more of a sense of community responsibility for other members of the society. Swedish citizens also generally believe that many organizations, including the government, should play a role in helping to benefit the community. They believe that traffic engineering, building codes, and product design should help ensure the safety of children, the elderly, and other potentially vulnerable populations. The joint efforts of many institutions have resulted in a large injury-prevention success story. The key to the success has been the societal approach to the promotion of safety.

LESSON: It takes a village to protect a child.

8.5. Country: The Netherlands

In the 1960s and 1970s urban walking and bicycling became increasingly difficult and dangerous in both the United States and Europe. The trend was to adapt the city to the car, giving top priority to car travel. Pedestrians were basically treated as motorists who had succeeded in parking their automobiles. In Europe pedestrian associations mobilized against this trend. One of the places where changes occurred to dramatically increase the appeal and safety of foot and pedal travel was the Netherlands.

In the past twenty-five years the Netherlands has made walking and cycling more attractive and safer. Policies have included traffic calming in residential neighborhoods by using physical barriers such as raised intersections, traffic circles, and speed bumps. Because the risk of pedestrian death in crashes rises from 5 percent at 20 mph to 45 percent at 30 mph to 85 percent at 40 mph, speed limits were reduced. The central city was also made more pedestrian friendly by creating extensive auto-free zones, wide and well-lit sidewalks, and pedestrian refuge islands for crossing wide streets.

The Dutch also doubled their already massive network of bike paths. In addition, the number of bicycle streets was increased; here, cars are permitted but bicycles have the right-of-way. A truly coordinated bikeway system now exists for everyday travel to practical destinations. By contrast, almost all bike paths in the United States are for recreation.

New suburban developments were also designed to provide convenient and safe pedestrian and bicycle travel. Residential developments typically included cultural centers and shopping, which could easily be reached on foot. By comparison, reaching U.S. strip malls is difficult and dangerous for both pedestrians and bicyclists.

In the United States, although over 40 percent of urban trips are less than two miles and 28 percent are shorter than one mile, the percentage of urban trips made by walking or cycling fell to 6 in 1995. By contrast, the percentage of walking or cycling urban trips in the Netherlands is 46 percent. Indeed, half the urban trips of Dutch ages 75 and over are by foot or bike.

"One of the biggest impediments to more walking and cycling is the appallingly unsafe, unpleasant, and inconvenient conditions faced by pedestrians and bicyclists in most American cities" (Pucher & Dijkstra 2003, 1511). How much more unsafe is it in the United States? Per mile, American pedestrians are six times more likely to be killed than Dutch pedestrians, and American bicyclists are three times more likely to be killed than Dutch cyclists. The differences were not always so stark. Between 1975 and 2000, even with declining rates of walking and bicycling, the absolute number of U.S. bike and pedestrian fatalities fell by less than 25 percent. By contrast, with increases in both walking and cycling, the total number of Dutch pedestrian fatalities fell 73 percent and bike fatalities fell 57 percent.

"The neglect of pedestrian and bicycling safety has made walking and cycling dangerous ways of getting around American cities. Walking and cycling can be made quite safe, however, as clearly shown by the much lower fatality and injury rates in the Netherlands" (Pucher & Dijkstra 2003, 1514). It is not that the Netherlands has more governmental intervention in the transportation sector than the United States. It is that their policies are designed to protect pedestrians and cyclists. And walking and cycling help promote other aspects of personal and public health. They help to reduce the likelihood of obesity, diabetes, and hypertension, and they help to alleviate traffic congestion, save energy, reduce air and noise pollution, and limit global warming.

LESSON: The issue is often not whether we should have
          governmental involvement; it is the extent to which
          governmental policies promote or detract from public
          health.

CHAPTER 9

Future Successes

INTRODUCTION

Despite many successes, injuries still exact a large toll on human life. In the United States in 2005 there were over 173,000 injury deaths; about 70 percent of these were unintentional injuries and 30 percent were intentional (i.e., suicide and homicide). There were also about 30 million nonfatal injuries that year serious enough to receive treatment at emergency departments. About 93 percent of these were unintentional injuries.

Injuries are the leading cause of death of young Americans. Indeed, in 2005 almost half of the deaths to children ages 10 to 14 and well over half of the deaths to adults ages 25 to 34 were due to injuries. Among those 15 to 24 approximately three-quarters of the deaths were injury-related, primarily motor vehicles and firearm deaths.

Fortunately most injuries can be readily prevented. In this chapter, I present a few examples of potential future success stories in preventing injury from motor vehicles, sports, and guns and preventing suicides. The issues chosen are not meant to be representative but to illustrate that there are many things that could be done, easily and cheaply, to reduce the number and severity of injuries.

For motor vehicle injuries the focus is on one problem: speeding; for sports injuries the focus is on baseball and softball injuries; for suicide the focus is on one suicidal site; the issue of firearm injuries is discussed more generally. In each area there is a discussion of only some of the many policies that could help reduce the problem.

Injuries continue to cause much pain, suffering, hardship, and economic loss. Prevention is typically both the most humane and cost-effective approach. There are many ways we can reduce the injury burden in the United States and throughout the world.

PROMISING POLICIES

9.1. Speed

Over three million Americans were killed on the highways in the past century. Each year in this country there are more than 11 million crashes. Crashes not only cause injury and property damage, but are the leading cause of urban traffic delays. Although there are not good data on speed in crashes, it is estimated that speeding is a factor in approximately 30 percent of motor vehicle fatalities.

Speed kills. It is so dangerous because it increases the stopping distance and the impact of the crash, both by the square of the speed. Table 5 gives the estimated stopping distance for an alert, capable driver, not under the influence of drugs or alcohol, on a dry road. These are therefore best estimates; a drunk driver on a wet road would take longer to stop. The table shows that under the best of conditions a motorists driving at 70 mph requires more than a football field to stop his or her vehicle. Another 85 feet are required if the vehicle is traveling at 80 mph. Averaging 80 mph rather than 70 mph saves only about five minutes on a fifty-mile trip.

The table also provides information on the relative impact of crashing into a deer or truck or brick wall at various speeds. In terms of energy or force of impact, it is about five times worse to hit a wall at 70 mph than at 30 mph. The impact of hitting a wall at 50 mph is almost three times worse than at 30 mph.

Government crash tests are conducted at 30 to 35 mph. A good seat belt and airbag will usually save your life in a 30 mph collision; they will not save your life in an 80 mph collision. It would take close to a football field for a motorist driving at 80 mph to reduce his or her vehicle speed to 30 mph.

A summary of the scientific literature concludes, "An enormous body of evidence consistently supports that the risk of crashing, being injured, or being killed, increases with increasing speed. There is no doubt that the dose-response curve is very steep—a little extra speed generates a lot more harm. . . . For fatalities, a one percent increase in speed appears to

TABLE 5

Speed, stopping distance, energy impact, and time saved

Speed (mph)	Approximate stopping distance (feet)	Relative impact energy	Time in minutes for 50-mile trip	Time savings by going 10 mph faster (minutes)	Stopping distance increase (feet) by going 10 mph faster
10	15	1	300		
20	40	4	150	150	25
30	75	9	100	50	35
40	120	16	75	25	45
50	175	25	60	15	55
60	240	36	50	10	65
70	315	49	43	7	75
80	400	64	38	5	85
90	495	81	33	5	95
100	600	100	30	3	105

increase fatality risk somewhere in the range 4% to 12%. . . . The lower value indicates that a 3% speed reduction reduces risk by 13%. This is larger than the reduction from frontal airbags" (Evans 2004, 216).

The 1974 reduction in the speed limit on U.S. interstate highways from 70 to 55 mph led to lower speeds on all roads. From 1973 to 1974 U.S. motor vehicle fatalities fell from over 55,000 to slightly more than 46,000. This drop of 16 percent was the largest yearly decline ever recorded in peacetime in the United States. The National Research Council attributed almost half of the drop to decreased speeds (National Highway Traffic Safety Administration 1984).

The increase in U.S. speed limits in the 1980s and 1990s led to an increase in fatalities. Studies by the Insurance Institute for Highway Safety and academic experts estimate that increasing the national speed limit for rural interstates in the late 1980s to 65 mph increased fatality rates on these roads by about 15 percent. The repeal of the national maximum speed limit in 1995 and the immediate increase in speed limits in twenty-four states increased deaths on interstates and freeways by another 15 percent ("Research and Statistics" 2007; Evans 2004; Greenstone 2002; Garber & Graham 1990).

Motorists often go faster than the speed limit. For example, in a study of Georgia teens, 80 percent reported having driven 20 mph over the speed limit (CDC 1994). In a survey of Maryland adults, a third admitted to driving 20 mph over the speed limit some of the time

(Lewis 2005). In a 2002 survey by National Highway Traffic Safety Administration (NHTSA) of over four thousand adults more than 80 percent reported speeding in the past month, and 12 percent reported going more than 20 mph faster than the speed limit sometimes or often on interstates (Compton 2005)

Still, speed limits affect speed. When the speed limit is raised, speed goes up. For example, New Mexico raised its speed limits to 65 mph on rural interstates in 1987, and the proportion of motorists exceeding 70 mph grew from 5 percent shortly after speed limits were raised to 36 percent in 1993. In 1996, when speed limits were further increased to 75 mph, more than 29 percent of motorists exceeded 75 mph; by 2003 55 percent of motorists exceeded 75 mph ("Research and Statistics" 2007).

Many policies can reduce the speeding problem in the United States, including changes in speed limits (hopefully designed to increase safety rather than simply to raise revenues through fines), changes in road design (e.g., traffic calming), and changes in enforcement (e.g., speed cameras). Here I briefly discuss three other initiatives: (1) standardizing and reducing speed governor settings for cars and trucks, (2) banning the sale of radar detectors, and (3) changing social norms regarding speeding.

Speed Governors   A quick and easy way to reduce some of the most excessive speeding is to standardize and reduce speed governor settings. All cars sold in the United States are equipped with electronic speed governors, which limit the maximum speed of the vehicle. These governors do not affect the acceleration of the vehicle, which is largely determined by horsepower. Speed governors are typically set between 110 and 160 mph. For example, in 2005 the governor of the Lexus IS300 was set at 144 mph, the BMW M3 at 137 mph, and the GMC Typhoon at 124 mph (Lewis 2005).

In the early 1970s the NHTSA issued a series of rule-making initiatives designed to regulate the maximum setting of speed governors at 95 mph. More than five hundred motorists wrote angry letters to the agency, asserting their right to drive faster than this, and the NHTSA ended its efforts.

There is no cost to standardizing and reducing speed governor settings. Although it is possible for motorists to change the settings, doing so requires some skill, and it is expected that few motorists would bother to make the change, just as few households change the setting of their hot water thermostats.

Setting the speed governor at 80 mph (police and emergency vehicles exempted) could reduce the danger from the most excessive speeders on highways, and also reduce the problem of high-speed chases, many of which involve stolen vehicles. High-speed police chases provide some exciting reality television, but they are dangerous for the pursued, the police, and innocent bystanders. More than one person a day is killed in these pursuits; over a third are innocent bystanders. It is noteworthy that most police chases are initiated as the result of traffic violations, not felony crimes ("Police Pursuit" 1992; Hill 2002).

Trucks traveling at excessive speeds are both frightening and dangerous. In March 2007, in a request for comments, the Insurance Institute for Highway Safety urged the NHTSA to require that speed governors on large trucks be set at 68 mph: "The United States lags behind Europe, Australia and Japan in requiring speed limiters on large trucks." For example, in 2002 the European Union mandated that speed limiters for large trucks be set at 56 mph (90 km/h; McCartt 2007, 3).

Radar Detectors   Radar detectors are vigorously marketed in the United States. Their sole purpose is to detect police radar in the area, thereby assisting motorists to speed illegally without getting caught. One study of radar detectors by the Insurance Institute for Highway Safety found that most users admitted to driving faster than they would have without their "fuzz busters." An observational study found that when speeding vehicles with radar detectors were exposed to police radar, speeds dropped by approximately 15 percent, but by one mile after exposure, nearly half of the reduction was recovered. This finding indicates "that radar detector users slow only briefly when alerted to police radar and that radar detectors are used primarily to avoid speed limit enforcement" (Teed et al. 1993, 136).

Radar detectors are banned in many developed countries, including Belgium, France, Germany, Norway, Sweden, Spain, Switzerland, and the Netherlands and most parts of Canada and Australia. They are illegal in all vehicles in Virginia and Washington, DC. Making them illegal throughout the United States could reduce excessive speeding at no cost.

Social Acceptability   Social norms affect behavior. For example, in some developed nations (e.g., Sweden, Switzerland) pedestrians rarely cross against traffic signals; in others (United States, United Kingdom, Canada) such behavior is common even though it is illegal to do so. In developed nations few drivers would consider driving on the sidewalk to save a few seconds; in many developing nations this practice is common even though it is illegal. "The cultivation of safe driving as habit seems a more productive approach than expecting drivers to be motivated by fear of consequences" (Evans 2004, 341).

One of the biggest obstacles to reducing the speeding problem in the United States is the social acceptability of speeding. Many people routinely speed, yet consider themselves law-abiding. Their behavior is not only common, but socially acceptable. Survey evidence confirms that, when asked, most drivers do not view driving 10 mph over the speed limit as wrong (Raymond 2002).

Moral judgments concerning speeding and drinking and driving diverged markedly over the past three decades. In the 1970s driving while intoxicated was illegal but was not considered socially unacceptable. After all, "social drinkers" were expected to have a few drinks at a restaurant or bar before they drove home. It wasn't until a social revolution, led by MADD, Students Against Drunk Driving (SADD), and others, that driving drunk began to be widely viewed as socially reprehensible behavior, which should be punished by stiff penalties. By contrast, speeding has remained largely socially acceptable. The difference is seen in the statistics: between 1982 and 2003, alcohol-related motor vehicle fatalities fell from over 25,000 to just over 17,000; in the same period, fatalities from crashes having nothing to do with alcohol increased 36 percent, from over 18,000 to over 25,000.

Prominent public officials can afford to admit, even brag about, a failure to comply with speeding laws. For example, a congressman and former governor of South Dakota boasted that his lead-foot driving led to twelve speeding tickets from 1990 to 1994. In 2003, while speeding through a stop sign, he killed a motorcyclist—for which he received a hundred-day sentence. "Nobody in public life could have boasted about driving while drunk, nor retained a driving license after a long series of drunk driving convictions. If the social norm and legislative response to speeding had been more like that to drunk driving, the motorcyclist would not have died and the politician would not have had his own life devastated by the crash" (Evans 2004, 343).

In 2007 the governor of New Jersey was on his way to his official residence to meet with the radio personality Don Imus and the Rutgers women's basketball team. His two-car motorcade was traveling at over 90 mph, more than 25 mph over the speed limit, with emergency lights flashing. Cars swerved getting out of the way, and one hit the SUV with the governor in the front seat. Disobeying New Jersey law, the governor was not wearing his seatbelt. His vehicle slid off the road and struck a guardrail. The governor sustained an open fracture of the left femur, eleven broken ribs, a broken sternum and collarbone, and a fractured lower vertebra. He had three operations on his leg and spent eighteen days in the hospital. He also issued a public apology. He began a public service announcement with, "I'm New Jersey Governor Jon Corzine and I should be dead." The announcement focused on the importance of wearing a seat belt. It did not mention the speeding.

A successful MADD-type public health campaign about speeding—indeed, about many risk-taking behaviors of sober drivers, including running red lights and stop signs, cell phone use, and text messaging—could save many lives.

9.2. Sports

Many modifications have made sports and recreation safer in the United States. For example, in football, rule changes such as those preventing spearing, clipping, chop blocking, and clothes lining have helped prevent injuries. In baseball, improvements to batting helmets and catching equipment have been beneficial. However, recreation is still not nearly as safe as it could be.

Injury control specialists like to imagine a world where games are designed so that safety is the top priority, a world where the main goals of sports are for individuals to participate, to acquire skills, to get exercise, to have fun, to engage in competition, to learn sportsmanship, teamwork, confidence, and perseverance—and not get hurt. Keep that perspective and read about sports injuries in the United States.

It is estimated that currently more than ten thousand Americans each *day* receive treatment in emergency departments for play-related activities (sports, recreation, exercise). Injuries are an important reason Americans stop physical activities. A major impediment to reducing the number of play injuries is the idea continually expressed by many coaches and parents that "injuries are part of the game" and that little can be done to reduce their occurrence. In actuality, most play injuries are preventable.

In this section we deal with two sports, baseball and softball, and mention only a few of the many policies that could reduce injury. It is estimated that over 20 million Americans play organized baseball each year, and the vast majority are youth under 20 years of age. Up to 40 million adults participate in organized softball.

Breakaway Bases   Sliding is a main cause of baseball and softball injuries, causing up to 70 percent of softball injuries. The more serious sliding injuries are ankle fractures, knee sprains, and shoulder dislocations.

What could be done to reduce sliding injuries? Making sliding illegal is a possibility, but such a drastic measure is unacceptable to most players. Recessed bases (e.g., home plate) are another alternative, but make it more difficult for umpires to determine whether the runner is safe or out. Better instruction on sliding techniques might help, but runners often do not follow these rules; in addition, most recreational players in the community don't have time for training. Many of these players are not in the best shape and are not expert players. The most cost-effective means of reducing sliding injuries is to modify the base.

Most bases are fixed, immovable, stationary objects. The base is bolted to a metal post and then sunk into the ground. By contrast, a breakaway base typically consists of two parts: a mat at ground level, which is attached to a post inserted into the ground, and a base that is snapped onto the mat. When a player slides into a breakaway base with great force, the base simply breaks away. It turns out that most sliding injuries could be eliminated with this one small change: the replacement of rigid bases with breakaway bases.

Roger Hall invented a Lego-type breakaway base after a friend broke a thighbone sliding into a stationary base and subsequently died from a blood clot that migrated to his lungs. Hall's base is a rubber mat with rubber thumbs on top over which the breakaway portion snaps into place.

Studies show the health benefits of such breakaway bases. For example, in a study involving softball, half of the fields used stationary bases and the other half used Hall's breakaway bases. Teams were assigned to playing fields on a random and rotating basis, so the same players were playing with both types of bases. After over 1,250 games, forty-seven sliding injuries had occurred: forty-five involved stationary bases and two involved breakaway bases. In other words, the new breakaway bases reduced the number of sliding injuries by 96 percent! In the following season breakaway bases were put on all the fields; in over 1,000 games there were only two sliding injuries. The directors of field supervisors reported that play was not significantly delayed due to the breakaway bases (i.e., they did not detach during routine base running) and the umpires had no additional difficulty with judgment calls (when the breakaway portion of the base did break away, the rubber mat that was flush with the infield surface was considered the base when determining whether the runner was safe or out).

Not only was there a 96 percent reduction in sliding injuries with the breakaway bases, but when injuries did occur they were less serious: direct medical costs per injury were half as much as those from the stationary bases. Based on the findings from this study, the Centers for Disease Control estimated that 1.7 million injuries could be prevented nationally each year, saving some $2 billion in medical costs (Janda 2003a, 2003b; Janda et al. 1988, 1990).

In a similar study of college and minor league baseball, breakaway bases reduced sliding injuries by 80 percent (Janda et al. 1993).

"Injuries are inherent in any recreational activity. Most base sliding accidents result from judgment errors of the runner, poor sliding technique, and inadequate physical conditioning. Break-away bases can serve as a passive intervention to modify the outcome of these factors. The use of break-away bases decreases injuries without player involvement or altering the play, excitement, entertainment, competition or interest in the game" (Janda et al. 1990, 635).

Breakaway bases are used in Little League and military and federal penitentiaries. They were used in the 2000 Olympics in Sydney, Australia. But most leagues in the United States still do not use them. In May 2007 the National Collegiate Athletic Association recommended that "the use of breakaway bases to prevent sliding injuries should be supported in collegiate baseball" (Dick et al. 2007, 192).

Aluminum Bats   In the 1970s aluminum bats were introduced into American baseball. Compared to the traditional wooden bats, metal bats can be made lighter and so swung faster; the sweet spot is much larger, and because of the so-called trampoline effect a hit ball travels faster and farther. Over time the manufacturers were able to make ever higher performance metal bats; for example, between 1994 and 1998 in Division I college baseball, home runs jumped from 0.69 per game to 1.06 per game.

Major league baseball has never allowed metal bats. It was felt that they would destroy comparability with the past in terms of batting records.

The main public health problem with metal bats is that faster balls pose a danger to fielders, in particular the pitcher. A batting cage study comparing the highest performing metal and wood bats found that the average difference in speed of a hit ball was approximately 9 mph

(Greenwald et al. 2001). With a metal bat, the pitcher loses precious microseconds in which to protect himself.

Jack MacKay, a former chief bat engineer for Louisville Slugger who helped design high-performance aluminum bats, has become a leading proponent for eliminating the metal bats. "This is the kind of technology you ought to be throwing at bin Laden, not some baseball pitcher. . . . We've over-engineered it. It's the worst thing I ever did. Aluminum bats and wood bats are not even in the same ballpark" (quoted in Keteyian 2002).

In 1999 colleges and high schools required manufacturers to redesign the aluminum bats so that when swung at the same speed as wood bats, the balls would not fly off faster. However, with a center of gravity closer to the bat handle, aluminum bats can be swung faster, and the balls hit off these bats still travel some 5 mph faster than off wood bats. Independent experts consider these speeds too fast (Adelson 2000; Ritter 2007).

Serious injuries from batted balls are rare, under two deaths per year. So it takes time, and good data, to show that any policy may be increasing the injury risk by even a factor of two. The University of North Carolina at Chapel Hill is conducting a study of college baseball games, analyzing injuries to pitchers from line drives. The comparison is between regular season games (aluminum bats) and summer league games (wood bats). Preliminary results from two seasons show that the aluminum bat injury rate was 2.6 times higher than the wood bat rate. But researchers say they need four more years of data to reach a definitive conclusion (Ritter 2007).

There appear to be no major health benefits to players from using metal bats, and a serious potential cost. If preventing injuries were the top priority leagues would not wait another four years for enough pitchers to become seriously injured before making a change. Indeed, many leagues have switched to wooden bats: the Cape Cod League, the Greater Boston High School League (after a pitcher was seriously injured by a batted ball), and, recently, New York public high schools. Yet the majority of organized high school and college baseball teams are still using aluminum bats.

Technology marches on, and new bats are being developed. When the goal of technology is performance rather than safety, people can get seriously hurt. For example, in softball, new titanium-based or composite-based softball bats are increasingly being used because they improve hitting. However, experimental field test data show that when these bats are used, "available pitcher reaction times are unsafe, which can lead to a higher injury risk potential" (McDowell & Ciocco 2006, 155).

In summary, many policies could help reduce baseball injuries. Aside from breakaway bases and wood bats, suggestions include a double-wide first base (part in foul territory) to reduce collisions between the fielder and the runner, face shields for batters, and screened-in dugouts to prevent players from being hit by foul line drives. Unfortunately few studies have actually examined the effects of such policies (Caine et al. 1996), and few evidence-based injury prevention programs for sports currently exist in the United States (Hootman et al. 2007). Many commonsense ideas that seem beneficial may actually have little or no effect. For example, studies find that certain types of softer baseballs, chest protectors, and breakaway bases do not offer much protection or reduce injury (Janda 2003b).

But good preventive measures can dramatically reduce sports injuries. A careful study of an established male soccer league in Sweden randomly divided twelve teams into two groups. The six teams in one group each received an intervention consisting of improved equipment, training, ankle taping, and other measures. The other six teams did not receive this injury-prevention intervention. At the end of six months the intervention teams had 75 percent fewer injuries (Ekstrand et al. 1983).

9.3. Suicide

Suicide Barrier at the Golden Gate Bridge   It is estimated that since its opening in 1937 almost fifteen hundred people have jumped to their death from San Francisco's Golden Gate Bridge. The bridge has become the leading suicide site in the world. At other places that attracted jumpers—the Empire State Building, the Duomo in Florence, St. Peter's Basilica, the Sydney Harbor Bridge, the Eiffel Tower, the Blood Street Viaduct in Toronto, and the Arroyo Seco Bridge in Pasadena—suicide barriers have been erected and have reduced the number of suicides to a handful or zero.

The fatality rate from jumping off the Golden Gate Bridge is 98 percent; only a couple of dozen jumpers have survived. Those who do often regret their decision—in midair. Said one, "I still see my hands coming off the railing. I instantly realized that everything in my life that I'd thought was unfixable was totally fixable—except for having just jumped." Said another, "My first thought was: What the hell did I just do? I don't want to die" (quoted in Friend 2003, 50).

Every jumper has his or her own story. One of the saddest was a "guy in his thirties, lived alone, pretty bare apartment. He'd written a note and left it on his bureau. It said, 'I'm going to walk to the bridge. If one person smiles at me on the way, I will not jump'" (Friend 2003, 59).

The current approach to preventing Golden Gate Bridge suicides is by using security cameras and patrols. One patrolman has coaxed more than two hundred potential jumpers away from the railing. He starts talking to a potential jumper by asking, "How are you feeling today?" followed by "What's your plan for tomorrow?" If the person doesn't have a plan, he says, "Well, let's make one. If it doesn't work out, you can always come back here later" (Friend 2003, 57).

The bridge has an allure for many potentially suicidal people, combining grandeur, glamour, beauty, and romance. Many people cross the Bay Bridge to jump from the Golden Gate; no one is known to have crossed the Golden Gate to jump from the less attractive Bay Bridge. As a suicide spot, the Golden Gate Bridge is also more accessible. It has a footpath adjacent to a low exterior railing, which is little deterrent. In 2005 a 75-year-old overweight woman was able to jump over the four-foot rail.

Death from jumping off the Golden Gate Bridge is sure, quick, and available. But there is nothing peaceful about a jump from the bridge. The fall takes about four seconds, then the body hits the water at 75 miles per hour, with the force of a speeding truck meeting a concrete building. Many jumpers die instantly.

Most people who commit suicide in the United States are suffering from major depression, bipolar disorder, schizophrenia, or drug and alcohol dependence. For those with mental illness, and those without, there are often precipitating crises, such as divorce, disease, or reversal of fortune. For a person in crisis the accessibility of the Golden Gate Bridge can be the tipping point between life and death. The people who kill themselves are overwhelmingly (87 percent) Bay Area residents.

Many organized attempts to support the building of an antisuicide barrier have failed, and lawsuits brought by the parents of suicides have been dismissed. In 1993 a man threw his 3-year-old daughter over the bridge and jumped after her. Even after this widely publicized tragedy a *San Francisco Examiner* poll found that the majority of residents opposed erecting a suicide barrier.

The three reasons given for opposing a suicide barrier are cost, aesthetics, and the belief that any barrier will be ineffectual, that people who really want to commit suicide will simply find another way. This reason is probably the most influential.

In 2004 a national survey of over 2,750 American adults asked what effect a suicide barrier might have had on the ultimate fate of the 1,500 people who have jumped to their death from the Golden Gate Bridge. Thirty-four percent of respondents believed that every single jumper would have found another way to complete suicide, and an additional 40 percent believed that "most" would have completed suicide using other means. The authors concluded that belief in the inevitability of suicide may be a political impediment to adopting potentially effective suicide prevention efforts (Miller et al. 2006).

The belief in the inevitability of suicide is unfounded. Studies of nearly lethal suicides, where the attempter expected to die and where death was highly likely, such as jumping in front of a subway, have found that fewer than 10 percent of the survivors ever go on to commit suicide (Owens et al. 2002). One study followed, for an average of over twenty-five years, more than five hundred people who were about to attempt suicide from the Golden Gate Bridge but were restrained. Fewer than 7 percent went on to commit suicide (Seiden 1978).

Installation of suicide barriers on other bridges has successfully reduced suicides from those bridges without appearing to increase suicides elsewhere (Lester 1993; Bennewith et al. 2007; Pelletier 2007). In another instance, removal of a bridge suicide barrier led to an immediate and substantial increase in the numbers of suicides from jumping from that bridge (Beautrais 2001).

Suicide experts agree that suicides are often impulsive, and the suicidal urge passes. During the danger period, helping to keep the individual out of harm's way can save his or her life. Restricting access to lethal means (e.g., don't leave loaded firearms around a potentially suicidal adolescent) is a sound public health strategy. This is why prisons and other institutions have suicide watches during times when an inmate is at high risk, taking away belts and other possible implements of self-destruction. When the period of great danger passes the prisoner is returned to a normal level of oversight. As the *San Francisco Chronicle* series on suicides from the Golden Gate Bridge observed, "The conclusion is inescapable: A suicide barrier would prevent deaths" (Guthmann 2005).

In the first decade of the twenty-first century there has been another groundswell of public, professional, and media support for the construction of a suicide barrier on the Golden Gate Bridge. A *New Yorker* article in 2003, a series of articles in the *San Francisco Chronicle*, an experimental film by Jenni Olson (*The Joy of Life*, 2005), and a documentary

film by Eric Steele (*The Bridge*) that captured on tape many of the suicides has helped reinvigorate the movement.

The idea is again being studied, this time by the Golden Gate Bridge
Suicide Deterrent Study. Constructing a suicide barrier would probably
save more than a dozen lives each year. Leaving the bridge without a
protective fence seems to imply a social sanction for those who would
jump. It would be far better if our policy choices would "provide clear
statements that we do not encourage self-destructive behavior—and
equally clear notice that we value constructive ways of dealing with the
pain and rage life contains" (Hendin 1995, 184).

9.4. Shootings

On a typical day in the United States in 2005 more than 275 people
were shot, and 84 died. The nonfatal injuries included traumatic brain
injuries and spinal cord injuries. There were more than one thousand
criminal gun uses per day, and countless batterers intimidated their intimate partners with firearms.

Compared to the other twenty-five populous developed democracies
(e.g., Australia, Canada, Germany, Italy, Norway, France, England, and
Japan), the United States has average rates of non-gun crime and non-
gun violence (e.g., assault, burglary, robbery, car theft). However, we
have many more guns, particularly handguns, and much more permissive gun control laws. We also have much higher rates of gun death. Our
firearms homicide rate is typically more than six times Canada's and
more than ten times that of Western Europe. We also have much higher
overall homicide rates than the other developed countries.

A study from the mid-1990s that focused on children found that our
violent death rate was far higher than that of other developed nations.
For children ages 5 to 14 the U.S. firearm homicide rate was seventeen
times higher than for the same age group in the other developed nations,
our firearm suicide rate was ten times higher, and our unintentional
firearm death rate was nine times higher. There was no difference in our
child non-firearm suicide rate compared to the other developed nations
(CDC 1997).

Guns make assaults and suicide attempts more lethal. More than a
dozen U.S. case control studies find that a gun in the home is a risk
factor for violent death (Hemenway 2006). These studies have focused
on homicide, suicide, or unintentional firearm death. The studies have
controlled for such factors as age, gender, education, community, living

alone, alcohol use, illicit drug use, and even psychiatric diagnosis. The suicide studies find that a gun in the home is a major risk factor for suicide death of the gun owner, the gun owner's spouse, and the gun owner's children.

Area-wide studies in the United States also find that in counties, cities, states, and regions with more guns there are more accidental gun deaths and more suicides and more homicides because there are more firearm suicides and more firearm homicides. A recent cross-state study of homicide controlled for rates of aggravated assault, robbery, unemployment, urbanization, alcohol consumption, and resource deprivation (e.g., poverty). States with higher levels of household firearm ownership had higher rates of firearm homicide and overall homicide. This relationship held for both sexes and all age groups. There was no association between state levels of household firearm ownership and non-firearm homicide (Miller et al. 2007a). A recent cross-state study for suicide controlled for poverty, unemployment, urbanization, mental illness, and drug and alcohol dependence. It found that in states with more guns there were substantially more suicides because there were more firearm suicides. This finding held for both sexes and all age groups. There was no relationship between state-level household firearm ownership and non-firearm suicide (Miller et al. 2007b).

The differences are large. To illustrate, Tables 6 and 7 compare the number of violent deaths to children ages 5 to 14 and to women in states with the highest versus the lowest levels of gun ownership in 2001–2004. The states with high gun ownership also have the more permissive gun policies. More states with high gun ownership are included so that the total populations are similar in these two groups of states (which allows for comparisons of numbers of deaths as well as death rates). As shown in Table 6, compared to children in states with low gun ownership, children in states with high gun ownership were more than twice as likely to be murdered with a gun, fourteen times more likely to commit suicide with a gun, and ten times more likely to die in an unintentional shooting. As shown in Table 7, compared to women in states with low gun ownership, women in states with high gun ownership were three times more likely to be murdered with a gun, eight times more likely to commit suicide with a gun, and six times more likely to die in an unintentional shooting.

There are scores of reasonable and feasible firearm policies that would not seriously restrict the ability of regular citizens to own firearms but could dramatically reduce our uniquely American gun

TABLE 6

Violent deaths of U.S. children (ages 5–14), 2001–2004

	States with high gun ownership	States with low gun ownership	Mortality rate ratio (High ownership: Low ownership)
Total population, children 5–14 (2001–2004)	21.0 million	21.7 million	
Homicides			
Gun homicides	97	41	2.4
Non-gun homicides	80	70	1.2
Total	177	111	1.6
Suicides			
Gun Suicides	68	5	14.1
Non-gun Suicides	106	74	1.5
Total	174	79	2.3
Unintentional firearm deaths	67	7	9.9

NOTE: The fifteen states with the highest average levels of household gun ownership (based on the 2001 Behavioral Risk Factor Surveillance System) were Wyoming, Montana, Alaska, South Dakota, Arkansas, West Virginia, Alabama, Idaho, Mississippi, North Dakota, Kentucky, Wisconsin, South Carolina, Utah, and Louisiana. The six states with the lowest average levels were Hawaii, Massachusetts, Rhode Island, New Jersey, Connecticut, and New York.

SOURCE: WISQARS (Centers for Disease Control and Prevention), http://www.cdc.gov/ncipc/wisqars/.

TABLE 7

Violent deaths of U.S. women (excludes the 9/11 terrorism attacks),

2001–2004

	States with high gun ownership	States with low gun ownership	Mortality rate ratio (High ownership: Low ownership)
Total population, women	75.9 million	82.4 million	
Homicides			
Gun homicides	1303	427	3.3
Non-gun homicides	1133	983	1.3
Total	2436	1410	1.9
Suicides			
Gun Suicides	1628	218	8.1
Non-gun Suicides	1932	1975	1.1
Total	3560	2193	1.8
Unintentional firearm deaths	109	19	6.2

SOURCE: WISQARS (Centers for Disease Control and Prevention), http://www.cdc.gov/ncipc/wisqars/.

injury problem. A public health approach to reducing our firearms problem would be based on three important concepts: (1) prevention is preferable to waiting until after the injury and violence have already occurred; (2) modifying the agent (the gun) and the environment are often more cost-effective than direct attempts to change individual behaviors; and (3) multiple strategies targeted at different risk factors are crucial.

Some policies could be focused on the individual gun owner. In virtually all other industrialized democracies—none of which has our serious firearm problem—gun owners need to be licensed (like car drivers) and handguns need to be registered (like cars). Both policies can reduce access of criminals to firearms and help police trace guns and solve crimes. In other developed countries gun owners are required to store their firearms safely, helping to reduce accidents and suicides. Waiting periods before the acquisition of a firearm are also common and may help reduce homicide as well as suicide rates. As the cartoon character Homer Simpson complained when faced with a waiting period to purchase a firearm, "But I'm angry now!"

Youth are at high risk of causing firearm injury. As the national legal age for purchasing alcohol is 21, the legal age for handgun ownership should also be raised to 21; this is currently the law in ten states ("Minimum Age" 2006). Alcohol is a risk factor for assaults as well as for bad driving. Although drinking is legal and driving is legal, we have wisely made it illegal to drive drunk, even if the driver has not broken any other law. Similarly, we should make the combination of heavy drinking and gun carrying illegal. Laws should also give police discretion to prohibit gun carrying by persons they know to be dangerous to the community.

Other policies could be directed at firearm manufacturers. I was at a meeting of the American Public Health Association in 1997 in Indianapolis. While waiting in line at a restaurant, a local resident reached down to pick up something off the floor, and a derringer fell out of his pocket. It hit the ground, went off, and shot two female delegates who were also waiting in line. Guns should not fire when dropped. Currently, however, we have virtually no national safety standards for American-made firearms.

Young children sometimes find a gun and shoot themselves and others. Handguns should be made child-proof; a toddler should not be able to fire a gun. As early as the late nineteenth century some firearms were deliberately made child-proof to reduce access by children.

In the United States a teenager who find his dad's pistol and takes out the magazine may believe the gun is unloaded; if he pulls the trigger he may kill his best friend. In many states such an act is considered a homicide since the teenager pulled the trigger intentionally. The easiest solution to these tragedies is to require that pistols have magazine safeties that prevent firing once the magazine has been removed.

Police are often unable to trace the firearms they seize. One reason is that criminals sometimes obliterate the serial number. Firearm manufacturers should be required not only to have unique identifiers for each firearm, but also to embed serial numbers in ways that are difficult to obliterate. Each handgun should also have ballistic microstamping that engraves a unique identifier into each fired bullet, permitting the easy matching of any bullet to a particular gun.

Some firearms and firearm accessories provide little social benefit but incur large potential social costs. Thus, except perhaps for bona fide collectors, the manufacture, sale, and possession of certain types of firearms and accessories should be prohibited; these include silencers, short-barreled shotguns, large-capacity ammunition magazines, and "gadget" guns that are difficult for metal detectors to identify and are disguised as innocuous items such as key chains, cigarette lighters, or pens.

The current firearm distribution system in the United States allows for easy access to firearms by criminals and terrorists. Some 40 percent of all firearm transfers in this country do not currently have background checks. Although there are tens of thousands of licensed firearm dealers, many people acquire firearms from private individuals at gun shows and flea markets, from newspaper ads, and over the Internet. All firearms transactions should be required to go through licensed dealers and be purchased from their retail premises, not from home kitchens, garages, or automobile trunks.

Criminals in states with strict gun control laws obtain their firearms from states with permissive laws. For example, 90 percent of firearms recovered in crime in New York City were originally obtained out of state. A national one-gun-per-month law, which would prohibit the sale of more than one handgun per month to any single individual, would eliminate much of the profit from gun running.

Licensing and registration also help reduce criminal access to firearms. A national handgun license card would make it more difficult for gunrunners to obtain fake identification documents and for violent persons to use temporary residence in another state to purchase firearms they could not buy in their home state. Registration of handguns would allow all legal firearm transfers to be efficiently traced. Current gun tracing typically provides information only about the initial retail sale. A registration system makes it less likely that an individual will act as a straw purchaser, someone with a clean record who buys guns for a criminal. Registration records make it easier to identify straw buyers, gunrunners, and rogue dealers.

Studies of inner-city youth consistently find that a substantial minority of boys has illegally carried firearms. The overwhelming reason given for carrying is for protection or self defense; they are afraid, largely because other teenagers (including youth gang members) are carrying firearms. Clearly, there is an arms race—in public health terms, a contagion effect—among these youth. Interventions that make access to firearms more difficult for inner-city youth can have a multiplicative effect, leading to large reductions in firearms violence.

One study asked adolescents, "Would you like to live in a world where it is easy, difficult, or impossible for teens to gain access to firearms?" The large majority chooses "impossible." Even among youth who have already illegally carried firearms, the majority typically wants it to be impossible for teens like themselves to obtain firearms (Hemenway et al. 1996; Hemenway & Miller 2004). Yet because they are afraid, they carry guns, making others less safe, more afraid, and more likely to carry firearms. We owe it to our youth to create a world in which they feel safe and are safe. The experience of every other developed country shows that we can do better.

Polls continually show that the large majority of Americans favor all the policies mentioned in this chapter. Indeed, the majority of gun owners, and even most members of the National Rifle Association, favor most of these policies. What is currently lacking is the will of enough people to stand up for our collective safety.

CHAPTER 10

Summary

INTRODUCTION

When I was a child I implicitly believed that it was the job of grown-ups to keep me safe. I thought that the organized games I played must have been designed to help me grow straight and strong and not get hurt. Perhaps this belief is a testament to my family and my community, to my innate optimism, or just to watching a lot of *Ozzie and Harriet, Father Knows Best,* and other TV shows in the 1950s. Of course, as I grew older I soon recognized that adults did not always act in ways that enhanced the interest of children or society.

Public health is a profession whose only goal is to promote the well-being of children and adults. The mission of public health is to "fulfill society's interest in assuring the conditions in which people can be healthy" (Institute of Medicine 1988, 4).

The focus of the clinical health professions (e.g., medicine, dentistry, nursing, optometry) is on treating individual patients; the focus of public health is on entire populations. Whereas patients tend to need medical care only some of the time (e.g., when they are ill), communities need public health all of the time. Some examples of public health are assuring that drinking water is safe, that pollution does not despoil the air and land, and that life-threatening diseases such as smallpox, polio, measles, tuberculosis, AIDS, and the Ebola virus are kept in check. Other public health concerns are reducing rates of substance abuse, heart disease, sexually transmitted disease, obesity, and violence. Public health also tries to assure good nutrition and safe work places, as well access to high-quality cost-effective medical care and rehabilitation.

Public health practitioners are idealists: they believe in progress and that they can help make the world a better place to live. But they are also pragmatists: they want to do what is most cost-effective to improve health and to reduce morbidity and mortality. The examples in this book highlight activities by public health professionals and others that have successfully reduced injuries and improved health.

Public health progress has often had to overcome the belief that nothing can be done about a problem until citizens improve their behavior. Traffic accidents, for example, were long considered solely the fault of the driver. Harry Barr, Chevrolet's chief engineer, articulated this viewpoint decades ago, before most cars had collapsible steering columns, seat belts, air bags, or anti-lock brakes: "We feel our cars are quite safe and reliable. . . . If drivers did everything they should, there wouldn't be any accidents" (quoted in Isaacs & Schroeder 2001, 28).

Historically the focus on finding a single cause of the accident limited the range of policies considered by decision makers. Not recognizing that injuries are rare events, police and highway personnel often argued that since the previous thousand drivers had not gotten into trouble at a specific crash location, the sole reason a particular person crashed must have been because he or she did something wrong. Without good data on exposure, these professionals were often unaware that the crash risk at a particular location was, say, 1 per 50,000 vehicles driving by, while the risk at a similar location, with better roadway design, was only 1 per 500,000. "In 1956, when as a senior medical student I first became interested in injury control, the major emphasis was still on single causes and on motivating, educating or regulating people to avoid the occurrence of crashes" (Waller 1994, 665).

Public health believes in individual responsibility, but only to the extent that the emphasis helps promote safety and well-being. An overemphasis on individual responsibility can be counterproductive. For example, until the second half of the twentieth century the focus of injury control was on preventing "accidents and the human misbehavior that precipitated them. Victim blaming and talk about 'accident proneness' were common" (Baker 1997, 369).

There is still too often a tendency to blame the victim, to emphasize the importance of personal responsibility. As Laurie Garrett, author of *Betrayal of Trust: The Collapse of Global Public Health*, claims, "America at the end of the twentieth century was reeling under the weight of its newfound libertarianism: the collective be damned, all public health burden and responsibilities fell to the individual" (Garrett 2000, 270).

Some personal responsibility is crucial for safety, and injury victims often did bizarre and stupid things. But the focus of the injury prevention field is to reduce injuries and violence, not to assign blame. And what the science shows is that usually the most cost-effective way to reduce injuries is to build a system that makes it difficult to make mistakes or to behave irresponsibly or unlawfully in the first place. In the second place, because humans inevitably will make some mistakes, behave irresponsibly, or ignore the law even in the most effective system, we must focus on making the environment safe. In most (but not all) of the success stories, it was not that people were more careful or better behaved, but that the system was a better one.

The approach is similar to that emphasized by human factors experts, who study human capability and develop systems with human limitation in mind: "Humans are essentially error-making and error-correcting entities. Since they pursue goals, they have sophisticated feedback mechanisms that measure deviations from the path to the goal. Error (deviation) is the input to the whole human decision-making process and cannot be designed out of the system. . . . The role of the designer is to enhance the possibility of error recovery and to produce an error tolerant system" (Hale & Glendon 1987, 33).

The public health and human factors approach is currently being applied to physician error. Instead of focusing on the doctor or nurse who made a mistake and punishing him or her, the emphasis is on designing a system in which it is highly unlikely that even a tired, harried medical provider will do something that leads to irreversible injury. The anesthesiology success story illustrates the benefits of that approach.

The public health approach needs to be applied more widely. Recently, as I was riding my bike home on Commonwealth Avenue in Boston, I was "doored." A parked motorist decided to open his door just as I was riding by, and I was knocked to the ground. I probably could make a case that it was his fault, but he didn't do anything deliberately wrong or stupid. Motorists are not trained to watch out for bicyclists when they open their car doors. Nor was it largely my fault; I was riding where it was safest to ride, as there was no bike lane. I try to ride on back streets, but this is not always possible. I try to watch for people in cars who might open the door, but this time I was not successful. Fortunately I was wearing a helmet, but I still sustained an injury. The real problem is that there is simply something wrong with the system; until improvements are made in roads to prevent such occurrences, such as by creating bike lanes, we can predict, and expect, many bicyclists to be doored each day in urban America.

The Success Stories

As individuals we all have successes in preventing injury. Getting enough sleep, eating healthy foods, exercising, not drinking to excess, driving defensively, wearing a seat belt, looking both ways before crossing the street—these all help reduce the likelihood that we will injure ourselves or others. The successes in this book are not about individual successes, but about public health successes, in which many people are directly affected.

The successes in this book include policies that have changed the human (the first column in the Haddon matrix), the agent of injury (the second column), or the environment (the third column). Policies that successfully altered human behavior to affect the pre-event phase of injury (Cell 1 of the Haddon matrix) include alcohol policies (e.g., minimum legal drinking age), graduated licensing, rules prohibiting stunting during the building of the Golden Gate Bridge, football rules outlawing tripping and crack-back blocking, and hunter orange requirements that lower the chance of being mistaken for game and getting shot. Policies that altered human behavior in ways that reduced the severity of injury during the event phase of injury (Cell 2) include getting people to buckle their seat belts and to wear helmets while riding a motorcycle or playing hockey. There may still be crashes and collisions, but with seat belts and helmets the likelihood of serious injury is reduced.

Many successes in this book changed the agent of injury. Injury control professionals generally prefer these more passive interventions because they do not require continual action, such as buckling up every time you get into a motor vehicle. Some of the successful policies focused on the pre-event phase (Cell 4): the third brake light in cars, child-resistant cigarette lighters, tap water preset at lower temperatures, and the banning of the short-handled hoe. Other policies have changed the agent of injury in ways that reduced the severity of injury during the event (Cell 5): air bags, collapsible steering columns, rollover protective structures, and flammability standards for pajamas.

Other successes in this book changed the environment. These are also passive approaches favored by injury control professionals. Requirements that landlords provide window guards (Cell 7: pre-event) and smoke detectors (Cell 8: event) helped parents prevent injury to children. Getting broken glass and aluminum cans off the sidewalk via bottle return laws reduced the likelihood of child injury (Cell 7: pre-event), as did making playground surfaces more forgiving (Cell 8: event). The built environment can make it more or less likely that children and adults will be injured, either unintentionally or intentionally; the Washington, DC, Metro was specifically and effectively designed to reduce injuries from violence.

Some successes in this book focus on the postevent phase of injury. Improvements in helicopter design reduced the likelihood of a serious fire after a crash (Cell 6). Improvements in medical treatment reduced the morbidity and mortality from wounds and other injuries (Cell 9).

There are many ways to increase safety. Many technological innovations were specifically targeted to reduce injury; these include inexpensive smoke detectors and improved ski bindings. Many rules for sports (e.g., hockey players must wear face masks and helmets) and for life (e.g., no buying alcohol before the age of 21) help reduce injury. Enforcement of laws often helps (e.g., random breadth tests, speed limit enforcement even for snowmobiles); so have requirements for the manufacture of various products (e.g., all cars must have collapsible steering columns; no leaded gas sales). Economic incentives have been used purposively to reduce injury; for example, taxing white phosphorus helped eliminate phossy jaw. Tort lawsuits also sometimes provide good incentives; for example, malpractice premiums for anesthesiologists helped spur major improvements in practice. Even government purchasing power has been used to provide a financial incentive for manufacturers to produce safer products, such as when the General Service Administration required that the cars it purchased must have air bags.

For many years the conventional approach to preventing unintentional injuries was to educate and exhort individuals, consumers and workers, to act safely. Thus in the United States we heard slogans such as "Don't smoke in bed" and jingles cautioning us to "Buckle up for safety." But there was little evidence that these national campaigns made much of a difference. For example, in response to the large-scale federal education program in the early 1980s seat belt use increased from 11 percent to only 15 percent (Gielen et al. 2006, 10).

Similarly, gun safety programs such as "Eddie Eagle" have been used in schools to teach children not to touch firearms. However, evaluations of such stand-alone educational programs typically show little effect on actual behavior. For example, the National Research Council's review of firearms education programs for children concluded that "there is little empirical evidence of positive effects on children's knowledge, attitudes, beliefs or behaviors" from such programs and that in fact, "for children, firearm violence education programs may result in increases in the very behaviors they are designed to prevent, by enhancing the allure of guns for young children" (National Research Council 2005). Human factors experts believe that "safety measures which are highly visible but largely ineffective should be treated with great suspicion" (Hale & Glendon 1987, 258). A problem with such measures is that they may give people a false sense of security and promote unsafe behavior; another problem is that such measures may hamper initiatives that could actually reduce the danger.

The scientific evidence indicates that it is generally easier and more effective to modify equipment and the environment than to educate or train individuals to always engage in safe behavior. It is not that educational programs focused on product users never work, but that, "despite the fact that fear is a strong motivator, the behavioral results of its use in health and safety are disappointingly small" (Hale & Glendon 1987, 279).

Effective educational programs need to be carefully designed; they work best when they are based on theory and are part of a comprehensive strategy. One positive benefit of education may be to increase public support for subsequent mandatory laws. Information on the benefits of seat belt use, for example, did little to change the number of people buckling up, but it did change attitudes toward the passage of seat belt laws, which have proved to be very effective in saving lives.

Rather than telling people what to think, information campaigns can effectively establish agendas, telling people what to think about. "Although there is little evidence that education alone works to change behavior, it can be a powerful initiator of and reinforcer for change" (Gielen et al. 2006, 12). Probably the most important injury prevention education in the twenty-first century will be "to influence employers, city planners, product designers, and decision-makers who have the authority to change the culture of safety" (Gielen et al. 2006, 2).

A second conventional approach for reducing both unintentional and intentional injuries is to increase enforcement: make it more likely that motorists who drive drunk will be caught and severely punished, and fewer motorists will drive drunk (Success Story 1.3). Similarly, make it more likely that individuals who assault others will face severe sanctions, and fewer people will commit assaults. However, scientific studies indicate that the severity of punishment is often less important than its certainty in deterring unwanted behavior. Although the United States has far higher rates of incarceration than other developed countries, we have average rates of crime and violence.

The key lesson from the science of injury control is that there are many types of policies besides education and enforcement that can cost-effectively reduce injury. Most of the success stories in this book are not directly about either increasing education or enforcement. The success stories help illustrate the fundamentals of the injury control approach. First, try to create a system that makes it more difficult for people to make mistakes (e.g., child-proof aspirin bottles that make it difficult for children to ingest multiple aspirin) or behave irresponsibly or unlawfully (e.g., architecture like the DC Metro that makes assaults less likely). Then, because some people will still make mistakes or behave inappropriately, the system should help ensure that few people are seriously injured (e.g., energy-absorbing steering columns, police body armor).

The injury control approach tries to get all possible stakeholders—industry, workers, insurance companies, standards writing associations, clergy, schools, architects, journalists, retailers, medical professionals, and injury survivors—to work together to prevent unintentional injury and violence. As the involvement of multiple stakeholders is better than the involvement of only one, so also will multiple interventions typically have far greater impact than single interventions. The examples from Boston, Harstad (Norway), and the Netherlands show the worth of the multiple stakeholder–multiple intervention approach in dramatically reducing injury.

The success stories highlight other important issues, such as the importance of good data and good research. Good research studies help garner support for interventions by documenting the size and scope of the problem, target interventions, and evaluate policies and programs to determine if they should be expanded or disbanded. For example, by obtaining data from ophthalmologists, Tom Pashby (Hero 4A, Success Story 4.4) documented the size of the eye injury problem in Canadian youth hockey, demonstrating the need for action; studies of teenage crashes showed the heightened dangers of night driving and driving with other adolescents in the vehicle, indicating the most effective rules for a graduated license system (Success Story 1.4); and evaluations of the fatal effects of lowering the minimum legal drinking age helped spur the U.S. government to raise the age to 21 (Success Story 1.1).

Some of the successes also illustrate the "law of unintended consequences." However, while most discussions of this so-called law provide

examples of good intentions leading to unintended negative consequences, in this book there are many examples of good intentions leading to unintended positive consequences. For example, increasing the
minimum legal drinking age not only reduced traffic fatalities of those
ages 18 to 20, but also seems to have reduced suicides (Success Story
1.1). Programs to reduce suicide in the Air Force had the unexpected
bonus of reducing intimate partner violence (Success Story 6.1).
Motorcycle helmet laws not only protected motorcyclists, but also dramatically reduced motorcycle theft (Success Story 1.6). And laws requiring deposits on glass bottles and metal cans, which were designed to
help clean up the environment, also helped reduce serious lacerations
among children (Success Story 4.8).

The success stories highlight the importance of governmental action.
Many safety improvements are the result of private enterprise respond-
ing to good market incentives to make less costly and safer products,
such as residential smoke detectors, improved ski boots, and avalanche
transceivers (Success Stories 2.3, 4.1, and 5.5). But most of the successes
in this book were due to smart government action, from mandating the
third brake light in cars to taxing dangerous products (Success Stories
1.8 and 3.1). Indeed, in many of the successes the government was
already buying cars; building roads, transit systems, and school playgrounds; and enforcing the law (Success Stories 1.10, 1.12, 6.4, 4.10, 1.2
and 4.12); the issue was whether the government would put sufficient
emphasis on public safety and act effectively (e.g., the Netherlands' success at protecting pedestrians and bicyclists, Success Story 8.5).

Finally, the stories illustrate the importance of good leadership. It
matters little whether the decision makers are public or private. The Air
Force success in reducing suicide (Success Story 6.1) and Alcoa's success
at preventing occupational injury (Success Hero 3E) show the power of
a committed, effective leader to lower injury rates. The Swedish success
demonstrates the huge improvements that are possible when effective
leaders of private and government organizations work in concert to protect the public (Success Story 8.4).

THE HEROES

What did the injury prevention heroes in this book have in common?
They all believed they could make a difference. They saw a problem—
specific serious injuries—and tried to prevent further suffering. These
heroes were humanitarians, with vision and energy. They were not to be

deterred. They believed they could make the world a safer place, and they succeeded. They worked tirelessly, often without financial reward.

These heroes came from all walks of life. Some were physicians (e.g., Robert Sanders, Barbara Barlow) and some had formal public health training (e.g., William Haddon, Janine Jagger), but there were also nurses (Florence Nightingale), scientists (William Redfield), businessmen (Paul O'Neill), clergy (Father Boyle), lawyers (Ralph Nader), housewives (Candy Lightner), and even an economist (John Andrews). It was not their training that mattered, but their passion.

Sometimes their key idea came from doing something different or seeing something from a different perspective. In automobile safety it was changing the question from "Who caused the accident?" to "What caused the injury?" (Hugh DeHaven, Bill Haddon); for needlestick injuries the question changed from "Why did you stick yourself?" to "What stuck you and how?" (Janine Jagger). Sometimes the key was seeing things in a different light: the idea that the direction of the wind could be different from the direction of the storm (William Redfield) or that lightning and electricity may be identical (Benjamin Franklin). Sometimes it was the decision to do something different: a surgeon who didn't wait for patients but went out of the hospital and into the community (Barbara Barlow), or one who decided to find out what happened to the patient en route to the hospital (Peter Safar). Sometimes it was just latching onto and really pushing for a good idea, such as a fire-safe cigarette (Andrew McGuire) or a line on the side of a ship (Samuel Plimsoll).

All these heroes faced obstacles and opposition, some from people or institutions that were tradition-bound and opposed to almost any change and some from powerful vested interests who believed they might be hurt by change. The road to success was long and difficult. Personal attacks were common. Samuel Plimsoll's reputation was besmirched and he was sued for libel; Ralph Nader was followed by private investigators; even Ben Franklin was accused not only of impropriety but of causing a Boston earthquake.

None of these heroes acted alone. Many people were involved in every success story in this book. But some people mattered more than others.

What are some of the lessons we might draw from this collection of public health (injury prevention) heroes? The first, and most important, is that a determined individual can make a difference, can save many lives. That is the principal message of this book.

Second is that it probably won't be easy; indeed, if it were easy the beneficial changes would probably already have happened. These individuals were not the first to perceive the problem, but often they were the first to really believe they could do something about it, even in the face of strong opposition. There are always obstacles, and there is virtually always opposition. It often seems incredible that there is such resistance; who could be against protecting children from the risk of serious burns or serious eye injuries? But there is resistance, typically fierce resistance. Success is usually slow in coming and it is hard won. It typically requires good data and good science. And it is rarely a complete victory.

Finally, the benefits are often seen only in the data (e.g., there are fewer children treated for serious burns). Sometimes one can see the benefits at an individual level (e.g., "I was in a collision and the air bag saved my life"), but not often (e.g., "I didn't get burned because there was no fire").

Who are the true American heroes? Baseball players? Actors who play violent heroes? Or people like Andrew McGuire and Paul Vinger who help prevent children from being seriously injured? How many of you had ever heard of either McGuire or Vinger before reading their stories in this book?

While we were leading our lives—eating, working, watching TV, or indeed, while we were sleeping—there were people who were working to make our lives safer. Mostly we don't know who they are, but they deserve our thanks. The heroes in this book are only a small sample of the people who have made a difference.

CONCLUSION

When I lecture about injury prevention, I often emphasize four points:

1. Injuries are a major public health problem.

2. Injuries follow predictable patterns and are often preventable.

3. Many interventions are possible; the trick is to pick the most cost-effective ones (usually modifying the product or the environment rather than trying to change human nature).

4. Individuals or small groups of dedicated individuals can make an enormous difference. As the anthropologist Margaret Mead is quoted as saying, "Never doubt that a small group of thoughtful, committed citizens can change the world; indeed, it is the only thing that ever has."

In J. D. Salinger's classic novel *Catcher in the Rye* Holden Caulfield's little sister, Phoebe, asks him what he wants to do when he grows up.

He responds, "I keep picturing all these little kids playing some game in this big field of rye and all. Thousands of little kids, and nobody's around—nobody big, I mean—except me. And I'm standing on the edge of some crazy cliff. What I have to do, I have to catch everybody if they start to go over the cliff—I mean if they're running and they don't look where they're going. I have to come out from somewhere and catch them. That's all I'd do all day. I'd just be the catcher in the rye and all. I know it's crazy, but that's the only thing I'd really like to be."

That is what public health is all about: preventing illness and injury. It is a good calling. Of course, instead of relying on Holden Caulfield to save one child at a time, public health workers want to assure that all children will be safe. They would build a fence at the top of the cliff, so the ambulance at the bottom would not be needed.

Appendix

Scientific Injury Studies

In 1985 *Injury in America*, a landmark report from the National Research Council and the Institute of Medicine, recommended a major national research program to address "serious, but remediable, inadequacies in the understanding and approach to injury as a health problem" (National Research Council 1985, 2). The report set out the rationale for conceptualizing injury prevention as a distinct field of study and recommended a major investment in injury research commensurate with the size of the problem. Following the recommendations of the report, Congress appropriated funds for an injury center at the Centers for Disease Control, helping to create the injury prevention field in public health (Institute of Medicine 1999). Since then the number of research studies in this area of public health has increased rapidly (Pless 2006), but the total amount of research—and funding for research—remains minuscule compared to the size of the problem.

The public health approach to injury prevention consists of answering four basic questions: What is the problem? What are the causes? What works to prevent this problem? And how do you get the programs that work implemented? To answer the first question, one needs to know what any good reporter would ask: Who? What? Where? When? How? Many cases need to be examined to answer these questions and to look for patterns. That first step is the essence of public health *surveillance:* collecting the data that help describe the extent and nature of the problem (Rosenberg & Hammond 1998).

In criminal justice parlance, *surveillance* is the term for monitoring the behavior of suspicious individuals. The public health meaning of surveillance is quite different; it refers to the systematic and continuing collection of health data essential for determining the nature of the problem, suggesting effective interventions, and providing information for policy evaluations. Collecting the same type of data over time and across sites is the key aspect of a surveillance system.

"You don't have to know where you are to be there. But you do have to know where you are to get somewhere else" (Foege 1996, xxv). A first step in addressing the epidemic of motor vehicle–related crashes during the 1960s was to start tracking all fatal motor vehicle crashes and collecting and analyzing detailed information about the circumstances and outcomes.

Researchers use surveillance and other data to investigate many issues in injury prevention. The small sample of articles that follows helps illustrate the wide variety of research topics in the injury field, as well as some of the methods currently employed.

Some studies are case reports (e.g., Car No. 1, an unusual burn caused by a car battery), designed to call attention to specific injuries being seen by medical care providers as well as to suggest treatments. Perhaps other physicians are seeing similar injuries, indicating that a systematic response to the problem may be necessary.

Some articles are retrospective reviews of medical records. One study (Car No. 2) found a substantial increase in serious injuries over time among children riding ATVs. Another study (Home No. 1) examined records from the Mayo Clinic and found that over three-quarters of the patients who sustained rib fractures as the result of coughing were women.

Some studies use surveillance data to determine levels of injury as well as risk and resiliency factors for injury, in part so that interventions can be better targeted. In one study (Violence No. 1) the authors used a CDC surveillance system and found that being a victim of dating violence was a risk factor for suicide attempts.

Some studies use interviews to elicit information. In a qualitative study (Work No. 1) more than two dozen Hispanic workers reported that the most common type of accident was falls, usually from a ladder, and the most common injuries were sprains and strains.

Some studies use written surveys to better understand the problem. Two important findings from a survey of Swiss basketball players (Play No. 1) were that over 15 percent of the players had already had dental trauma, yet only 1 percent of the over three hundred players interviewed wore mouth guards. A questionnaire completed by Indian Air Force personnel concerning injuries sustained during ejection indicated that practicing ejection drills and assuming correct posture were important to reduce the risk of injury (Work No. 2).

In case-control studies researchers begin by identifying a group of subjects known to have the outcome of interest (the cases). The controls are subjects who would have been counted as cases if they had the outcome of interest. In one study (Home No. 2) the cases were firearms that had been used by a young person in a suicide attempt or to unintentionally injury someone, and controls were firearms in households that had at least one young person. Guns stored unloaded and locked up substantially reduced the likelihood of firearm injury.

Some studies use natural experiments to determine the effects of various courses of action. In 2003, a tornado struck an Oklahoma City commuter bus. Some passengers evacuated to a ditch, while others remained on the bus (Nature No. 1). The researchers reported that examining the resulting injuries supported the recommendation to immediately evacuate the motor vehicle and lie in a low-lying area away from the vehicle when caught in a tornado.

Some studies use data to evaluate programs and policies to see what is and is not working, whether the policy should be changed, and how it can be made better. One study (Violence No. 2) compared more than one thousand cases (those exposed to an antibullying program) with controls (those not exposed) and found large improvements in achievement test scores associated with this simple, low-cost program.

Some articles summarize the literature, using meta-analyses or methods of systematically reviewing the research evidence. In one of these (Work No. 3) the author concluded that excessive verbal abuse in the emergency department is a global phenomenon, but it is much more likely for a patient to come in carrying a weapon in the United States than in the United Kingdom.

All these studies add to our knowledge and allow us to individually make better decisions about our own lives and to collectively make better policies to reduce the likelihood of serious injury.

SAMPLE ARTICLES

Car

1. Nisanci M., Sengezer M., Durmus M. 2005. An unusual burn injury caused by a car battery. *J Burn Care Rehabil.* 26:379–81.
2. Kelleher C.M., Metze S.L., Dillon P.A., Mychaliska G.B., Keshen T.H., Foglia R.P. 2005. Unsafe at any speed: Kids riding all-terrain vehicles. *J Pediatr Surg.* 40:929–34.
3. Pobereskin L. 2005. Whiplash following rear end collisions: A prospective cohort study. *J Neurol Neurosurg Psychiatry.* 76:1146–51.
4. Jones-Alexander J., Blanchard E.B., Hickling E.J. 2005. Psychophysiological assessment of youthful motor vehicle accident survivors. *Appl Psychophysiol Biofeedback.* 30:115–23.
5. Kamimura N., Kakeda K., Kitamura Y., Sanada J., Ikeda M., Inoue S. 2005. Dementia and driving: Present status of drivers with dementia and response of their family's care in Japan. *No To Shinkei.* 57:409–14.
6. Hakamies-Blomqvist L., Wiklund M., Henriksson P. 2005. Predicting older drivers' accident involvement: Smeed's law revisited. *Accid Anal Prev.* 37:675–80.
7. Matsui Y. 2005. Effects of vehicle bumper height and impact velocity on type of lower extremity injury in vehicle-pedestrian accidents. *Accid Anal Prev.* 37:633–40.

Home

1. Hanak V., Hartman T.E., Ryu J.H. 2005. Cough-induced rib fractures. *Mayo Clin Proc.* 80:879–82.
2. Grossman D.C., Mueller B.A., Riedy C., Dowd M.D., Villaveces A., Prodzinski J., Nakagawara J., Howard J., Thiersch N., Harruff R. 2005. Gun storage practices and risk of youth suicide and unintentional firearm injuries. *JAMA.* 293:740–41.
3. Alias A., Krishnapillai R., Teng H.W., Abd Latif A.Z., Adnan J.S. 2005. Head injuries from fan blades among children. *Asian J Surg.* 28:168–70.
4. Moustaki M., Pitsos N., Dalamaga M., Dessypris N., Petridou E. 2005. Home and leisure activities and childhood knee injuries. *Injury.* 36:644–50.

5. Landi F., Onder G., Cesari M., Barillaro C., Russo A., Bernabei R. 2005. Psychotropic medications and risk for falls among community-dwelling frail older people: An observational study. *J Gerontol B Psychol Sci Soc Sci.* 60:622–26.

Work

1. Salazar M. K., Keifer M., Negrete M., Estrada F., Synder K. 2005. Occupational risk among orchard workers: A descriptive study. *Fam Community Health.* 28:239–52.
2. Taneja N., Pinto L. J., Dogra M. 2005. Aircrew ejection experience: Questionnaire responses from 20 survivors. *Aviat Space Environ Med.* 76:670–74.
3. Ferns T. 2005. Violence in the accident and emergency department: An international perspective. *Accid Emerg Nurs.* 13:180–85.
4. Wang J., Pillay A., Kwon Y. S., Wall A. D., Loughran C. G. 2005. An analysis of fishing vessel accidents. *Accid Anal Prev.* 37:1019–24.
5. Jovanovic J., Jovanovic M., Lekovic S., Arizanovic A., Adamovic S. 2005. Occupational accidents in Serbian industries in transition. *Cent Eur J Public Health.* 13:66–73.
6. Poupon M., Caye N., Duteille F., Pannier M. 2005. Cement burns: Retrospective study of 18 cases and review of the literature. *Burns.* 31:910–14.
7. Haslam R. A., Hide S. A., Gibb A. G. F., Gyi D. E., Pavitt T., Atkinson S., Duff A. R. 2005. Contributing factors in construction accidents. *Appl Ergon.* 36:401–15.

Play

1. Perunski S., Lang B., Pohl Y., Filippi A. 2005. Level of information concerning dental injuries and their prevention in Swiss basketball: A survey among players and coaches. *Dent Traumatol.* 21:195–200.
2. Chen H. Y., Sheu M. H., Tseng L. M. 2005. Bicycle-handlebar hernia: A rare traumatic abdominal wall hernia. *J Chin Med Assoc.* 68:283–85.
3. Turgut A. T., Kosar U., Kosar P., Karabulut A. 2005. Scrotal sonographic findings in equestrians. *J Ultrasound Med.* 24:911–17.
4. Wiesler E. R., Lumsden B. 2005. Golf injuries of the upper extremity. *J Surg Orthop Adv.* 14:1–7.
5. Shields B. J., Fernandez S. A., Smith G. A. 2005. Comparison of mini-trampoline and full-sized trampoline-related injuries in the United States, 1990–2002. *Pediatrics.* 116:96–103.

Nature

1. Comstock R. D., Mallonee S. 2005. Get off the bus: Sound strategy for injury prevention during a tornado? *Prehosp Disaster Med.* 20:189–92.
2. de Roodt A. R., Salomon O. D., Orduna T. A., Robles Ortiz L. E., Paniagua Solis J. F., Alagon Cano A. 2005. Poisoning by bee sting. *Gac Med Mex.* 141:215–22.

3. Keuster T. D., Lamoureux J., Kahn A. 2005. Epidemiology of dog bites: A Belgian experience of canine behavior and public health concerns. *Vet Journal.* 172:482–87.
4. Ritter E. K., Levine M. 2005. Bite motivation of sharks reflected by the wound structure on humans. *Am J Forensic Med Pathol.* 26:136–40.
5. Dwyer J. R. 2005. Lightning: A bolt out of the blue. *Scientific American.* 292(5):64–71.

Violence

1. Bae S., Ye R., Chen S., Rivers P. A., Singh K. P. 2005. Risky behaviors and factors associated with suicide attempt in adolescents. *Arch Suicide Res.* 9:193–202.
2. Fonagy P., Twemlow S. W., Vernberg E., Sacco F. C., Little T. D. 2005. Creating a peaceful school learning environment: The impact of an anti-bullying program on educational attainment in elementary schools. *Med Sci Monit.* 11:CR317–25.
3. Barnes P. M., Norton C. M., Dunstan F. D., Kemp A. M., Yates D. W., Sibert J. R. 2005. Abdominal injury due to child abuse. *Lancet.* 366:234–35.
4. Foa E. B., Cahill S. P., Boscarino J. A., Hobfoll S. E., Lahad M., McNally R. J., Solomon Z. 2005. Social, psychological and psychiatric interventions following terrorist attacks: Recommendations for practice and research. *Neuropsychopharmacology.* 30:1806–17.
5. Teplin L. A., McClelland G. M., Abram K. M., Mileusnic D. 2005. Early violent death among delinquent youth: A prospective longitudinal study. *Pediatrics.* 115:1586–93.
6. Shalev A. Y., Freedman S. 2005. PTSD following terrorist attacks: A prospective evaluation. *Am J Psychiatry.* 162:1188–91.
7. Amar A. F., Gennaro S. 2005. Dating violence in college women: Associated physical injury, healthcare usage and mental health symptoms. *Nurs Res.* 54:235–42.
8. Marshall A. D., Panuzio J., Taft C. T. 2005. Intimate partner violence among military veterans and active duty servicemen. *Clin Psychol Rev.* 25:862–76.
9. Funk J. B. 2005. Children's exposure to violent video games and desensitization to violence. *Child Adolesc Psychiatr Clin N Am.* 14:387–404.

Medical Treatment

1. Tan H. B., Solan J. P., Barlow I. F. 2005. Improvement in initial survival of spinal injuries: A 10 year audit. *Injury.* 36:941–45.
2. Goans R. E., Wald N. 2005. Radiation accidents with multi-organ failure in the United States. *Br J Radiol.* (Suppl 27):41–46.
3. Townes D. A. 2005. Winderness medicine: Strategies for provision of medical support for adventure racing. *Sports Med.* 35:557–64.
4. Weinberg L., Steele R. G., Pugh R., Higgins S., Herbert M., Story D. 2005. The pregnant trauma patient. *Anaesth Intensive Care.* 33:167–80.

References

PREFACE

Houston D. J., Richardson L. E. 2008. Motorcyclist fatality rates and mandatory helmet-use laws. *Accid Anal Prev.* 40:200–208.

Chenier T. C., Evans L. 1987. Motorcyclist fatalities and the repeal of mandatory helmet laws. *Accid Anal Prev.* 19:133–39.

Mathews D. 2002. *War Prevention Works: 50 Stories of People Resolving Conflict.* Oxford: Oxford Research Group.

INTRODUCTION

Evans R. G., Barer M. L., Marmor T. R., eds. 1994. *Why Are Some People Healthy and Others Not? The Determinants of Health of Populations.* New York: Aldine de Gruyer.

Winslow C. E. A. 1923. *The Evolution and Significance of the Modern Public Health Campaign.* New Haven: Yale University Press.

Haines H. H. 1997. Nominal medicalization and scientific legitimacy in the pubic health approach to violence. In *Proceedings of the Society for the Study of Social Problems Annual Meeting, Toronto, Canada.* Knoxville, TN: Society for the Study of Social Problems.

Institute of Medicine. 1999. *Reducing the Burden of Injury.* Washington, DC: National Academy Press.

John Snow, father of epidemiology. 2005. UCLA Department of Epidemiology website. http://www.ph.ucla.edu/epi/snow.html. Updated June 2005. Accessed September 25, 2005.

1. CAR

Introduction

Evans P. 2004. *Traffic Safety*. Bloomfield Hills, MI: Science Serving Society.

Crandall R., Gruenspecht H., Keeler T., Lave L. 1986. *Regulating the Automobile*. Washington, DC: Brookings Institution.

Elvik R. 2001. Area-wide urban traffic calming schemes: A meta-analysis of safety effects. *Accid Anal Prev.* 33:327–36.

Centers for Disease Control and Prevention. 1999. Motor vehicle safety: A twentieth century public health achievement. *Morbidity and Mortality Weekly Report,*May 14, 369–74. Reprinted in *JAMA,* 1999; 281:2080–82.

Waller P. F. 2002. Challenges in motor vehicle safety. *Annu Rev Public Health.* 23:93–113.

1.1. Minimum Legal Drinking Age

Shultz R. A., Elder R. W., Sleet D. A., et al. 2001. Reviews of the evidence regarding interventions to reduce alcohol-impaired driving. *Am J Prev Med.* 21(4S):66–88.

Wagenaar A. C., Toomey T. L. 2002. Effects of minimum drinking age laws: Review and analyses of the literature from 1960 to 2000. *J Stud Alcohol.* 14:206–25.

Voas R. B., Tippetts A. S., Fell J. C. 2003. Assessing the effectiveness of legal drinking age and zero tolerance laws in the United States. *Accid Anal Prev.* 35:579–87.

Birckmayer J., Hemenway D. 1999. Minimum-age drinking laws and youth suicide, 1970–1990. *Am J Public Health.* 89:1365–68.

1.2. Random Breath Testing

Homel R. J. 1990. Random breath testing the Australian way: A model for the United States? *Alcohol Health Res World.* Winter.

Elder R. W., Shults R. A., Sleet D. A., Nichols J. L., Zaza S., Thompson R. S. 2002. Effectiveness of sobriety checkpoints for reducing alcohol-involved crashes. *Traffic Inj Prev.* 3:266–74.

Evans L. 2004. *Traffic Safety*. Bloomfield Hills, MI: Science Serving Society.

1.3. Increased Penalties for Drunk Driving

Nagata T., Setoguchi S., Hemenway D., Perry M. J. 2008. Effectiveness of a law to reduce alcohol-impaired driving in Japan. *Inj Prev.* 14:19–23.

Imai H. 2003. The new traffic law and reduction of alcohol related fatal crashes in Japan. *Inj Prev.* 9:382.

1.4. Graduated Driver's Licenses

Waller P. F. 2003. The genesis of GDL. *J Safety Res.* 34:17–23.

Evans L. 2004. *Traffic Safety*. Bloomfield Hills, MI: Science Serving Society.

Shope J. T., Molnar L. J. 2004. Michigan's graduated driver licensing program: Evaluation of first four years. *J Safety Res.* 35:337–44.

Shope J. T., Molnar L. J. 2003. Graduated driver licensing in the United States: Evaluation results from the early programs. *J Safety Res.* 34:63–69.

Rice T. M., Peek-Asa C., Kraus J. F. 2004. Effect of the California graduated driver licensing program. *J Safety Res.* 35:375–81.

Chen L. H., Baker S. P. 2006. Graduated driver licensing and fatal crashes of 16-year-old drivers: A national evaluation. *Pediatrics.* 118:55–62.

Shope J. T. 2007. Graduated driver licensing: Review of evaluation results since 2002. *J Safety Res.* 38:165–75.

1.5. Seat Belt Use

Haseltine P. W. 2001. Seat belt use in motor vehicles: The U.S. experience. In *Proceedings of the 2001 Seat Belt Summit: Policy Options for Increasing Seat Belt Use in the United States in 2001 and Beyond, January 11–13*. Arlington, VA: Automotive Coalition for Traffic Safety.

Graham, J. D. 1989. *Auto Safety: Assessing America's Performance*. Dover, MA: Auburn House.

1.6. Helmet Laws

Tsai M. C., Hemenway D. 1999. Effect of the mandatory helmet law in Taiwan. *Inj Prev.* 5:290–91.

Chiu W. T., Kuo C. Y., Hung C. C., et al. 2000. The effect of the Taiwan motorcycle helmet use law on head injuries. *Am J Public Health.* 90:793–96.

Mayhew P. M., Clarke R. V., Elliott D. 1989. Motorcycle theft, helmet legislation and displacement. *Howard Law J.* 28:1–8.

1.7. Child Safety Seats

Decker M. D., Dewey M. J., Hutcheson R. H. Jr., Schaffner W. 1984. The use and efficacy of child restraint devices: The Tennessee experience, 1982 and 1983. *JAMA.* 252:2571–75.

Kalbfleisch J., Rivara F. 1989. Principles in injury control: Lessons to be learned from child safety seats. *Pediatr Emerg Care.* 5:131–34.

Editorial. 1998. Celebrating the first child passenger safety law. *Safe Ride News.* Spring: 2.

1.8. Third Break Light

National Highway Traffic Safety Administration. 2006. *Traffic Safety Facts 2005*. DOT HS-810–616. Washington, DC: U.S. Department of Transportation, December.

Farmer C. M. 1996. Effectiveness estimates for center high mounted stop lamps: A six-year study. *Accid Anal Prev.* 28:201–8.

Kahane C. J. 1998. The long-term effectiveness of center high mounted stop lamps in passenger cars and light trucks. NHTSA Technical Report Number DOT HS 808–696. http://www.nhtsa.dot.gov/cars/rules/regrev/evaluate/808696.html. Updated March 1998. Accessed March 10, 2008.

1.9. Energy-Absorbing Steering Columns

National Highway Traffic Safety Administration. 1981. *An Evaluation of Federal Motor Vehicle Safety Standards for Passenger Car Steering Assemblies.* NHTSA Report Number DOT HS 805–705. Washington, DC: U.S. Dept. of Transportation, January.
Evans, L. 2004. *Traffic Safety.* Bloomfield Hills, MI: Science Serving Society.

1.10. Government Purchase of Air Bags

Hemenway D. 1989. Government procurement leverage. *J Public Health Policy.* 10:123–25.
Graham J. D. 1989. *Auto Safety: Assessing America's Performance.* Dover, MA: Auburn House.

1.11. Unleaded Gasoline

Reyes J. W. 2007. Environmental policy as social policy? The impact of childhood lead exposure on crime. *B.E. J Econ Anal Policy.* 7(1) Article 51.
Rosner D, Markowitz G. 1985. A gift of god? The public health controversy over leaded gasoline during the 1920s. *Am J Public Health.* 75:344–52.
U.S. Environmental Protection Agency. 2000. *America's Children and the Environment: A First View of Available Measures.* EPA 240/R-00–006. Washington, DC: Office of Children's Health Protection.
Kitman J. L. 2000. The secret history of lead: A special report. *The Nation.* March 20. http://www.thenation.com/doc.mhtml?i=20000320&c=1&s=kitman. Accessed March 2008.

1.12. Roundabouts

Elvik R., Vaa T. 2004. *The Handbook of Road Safety Measures.* Boston: Elsevier.
Persaud B., Retting R., Garder P., Lord D. 2001. Observational before-after study of the safety effects of U.S. roundabout conversions using the Empirical Bayes method. TRB paper 01–0562 presented at the 80th annual meeting of the Transportation Research Board, Washington, DC, January.
Bendtsen H. 1992. Rundkorsler reducerer luftforureningen. *Dansk Vejtidsskrift.* 10:34.
Varhelyi A. 1993. Minirondeller. *Energi-ofch miljoeffekter.* TFB-rapport 1993–6.

1.13. Guardrails

Short D., Robertson L. S. 1998. Motor vehicle death reductions from guardrail installation. *J Trans Engineering.* 124:501–2.

1.14. Crash Cushions

Wendling W. H. 1996. Roadside safety milestones. In Proceedings from the Semisesquicentennial Transportation Conference, Center for Transportation

Research and Education, Iowa State University, Ames. http://www.ctre.iastate.edu/pubs/semisesq/session1/wendling. Updated May 1996. Accessed July 2005.

Elvik R., Vaa T. 2004. *The Handbook of Road Safety Measures*. Boston: Elsevier.

Elvik R. 1995. The safety value of guardrails and crash cushions: A meta-analysis of evidence from evaluation studies. *Accid Anal Prev.* 27:523–49.

Forgiving roadsides. 1998. European Transport Safety Council website. http://www.etsc.be/documents/bri_road5.pdf. Updated 1998. Accessed July 2005.

Griffin L. I. III. 1984. How effective are crash cushions in reducing deaths and injuries? *Public Roads.* 47(4):132–34.

1.a. Hugh DeHaven

Pless, I. B. 2000. Editor's comment. *Inj Prev.* 6:62.

Winston F. K. 2000. The beginning of injury science. *Inj Prev.* 6:62.

Aldman B. 2005. The early history of the lap and shoulder, three-point safety belt. Autoliv website. http://www.autoliv.com/Appl_ALV/alvweb.nsf/Files/Belthist/$file/Belthist.pdf. Accessed March 7, 2005.

Hugh DeHaven. 2005. National Safety Council's Safety and Health Hall of Fame International website. http://www.shhofi.org/inductees/Bios/dehaven90.htm. Accessed March 7, 2005.

DeHaven H. 1942. Mechanical analysis of survival in falls from heights of fifty to one hundred and fifty feet. *War Medicine.* 2:586–96.

1.b. John Paul Stapp

Spark N. T. 2003. Fastest man on earth: The story of John Paul Stapp. *Airpower.* July 1.

Thomas D. E. 2000. Fastest man on earth, Colonel John Paul Stapp dies at 89; had connection to Roswell incident, Murphy's law. *Skeptical Inquirer.* March.

1.c. William Haddon

Christoffel T., Gallagher S. S. 1999. *Injury Prevention and Public Health: Practical Knowledge, Skills and Strategies*. Gaithersburg, MD: Aspen.

Robertson L. S. 1998. *Injury Epidemiology: Research and Control Strategies*. 2nd ed. New York: Oxford University Press.

ICADTS Reporter. 1999. International Council on Alcohol, Drugs and Traffic Safety website. http://www.icadts.org/reporter/v1on3.html. Updated Summer 1999 (10)3. Accessed March 2008.

Baker S. P. 1997. Advances and adventures in trauma prevention. *J Trauma.* 42:369–73.

O'Neill B. 2002. Accidents or crashes: Highway safety and William Haddon, Jr. *Contingencies.* January/February: 30–32.

Robertson L. S. 1983. *Injuries: Causes, Control Strategies and Public Policy*. Lexington, MA: Lexington Books.

National Committee for Injury Prevention and Control. 1989. Injury preven-
    tion: Meeting the Challenge. *Am J of Prev Med.* 5:4–8.

1.d. Ralph Nader

Marcello P. C. 2004. *Ralph Nader: A Biography.* Westport, CT: Greenwood Press.
Bollier D. 2004. Citizen Action. Ralph Nader website. http://www.nader.
    org/index.php?/archives/7-Citizen-Action-and-Other-Big-Ideas-By-David-
    Bollier-Chapter-One-The-Beginnings.html. Updated January 8, 2004.
    Accessed March 2008.

1.e. Seymour Charles and Robert Sanders

Pediatrician honored for fifty years of dedication to public health issues and
    child safety. 2005. Saint Barnabas Health Care System website. http://
    www.sbhcs.com/hospitals/saint%5Fbarnabas/press/pre2002/pediatrician.html.
    Updated June 2005. Accessed March 2008.
Seymour C. 2005. Father of child passenger safety dies: Seymour Charles, MD.
    Safe Ride News website. http://www.saferidenews.com/back_issues/2002/
    02SeptOct.pdf. Updated June 2005. Accessed March 2008.
Shelness A., Charles S. 1975. Children as passengers in automobiles: The neg-
    lected minority on the nation's highways. *Pediatrics.* 56(2):271–84.
Dewey-Kollen J. 2005. Pediatricians as CPS advocates. Safe Ride News website.
    http://www.saferidenews.com/back_issues/2003/03JulAug.pdf. Updated
    June 2005. Accessed March 2008.
Safety award renamed in honor of Dr. Robert Sanders. 2007. General Motors
    website. http://www.gm.com/company/gmability/safety/news_issues/releases/
    safe_kids_102306.html. Updated October 2007. Accessed February 2007.

1.f. Candy Lightner

Frantzich S. E. 2005. *Citizen Democracy: Political Activists in a Cynical Age.*
    2nd ed. New York: Rowman & Littlefield.
Creamer B. 1984. Candy Lightner's MADD: An organization formed of her
    anger and anguish. *Honolulu Advertiser,* February 10.
National Highway Traffic Safety Administration. 2002. *Traffic Safety Facts 2001.*
    DOT HS-809-484. Washington, DC: U.S. Department of Transportation,
    December.
Weed F. J. 1993. The MADD queen: Charisma and the founder of Mothers
    Against Drunk Driving. *Leadership Quarterly.* 4:329–46.

2. HOME

Introduction

American Medical Association. 2005. Preventing common household accidents.
    Medical Library. http://www.medem.com/MedLB/article_detaillb.cfm?
    article_ID=ZZZ5LGJLK9C&sub_cat=104. Accessed July 2005.

Baker S. P., Fisher R. S. 1980. Childhood asphyxiation by choking or suffocation. *JAMA*. 244:1343–46.

2.1. Child-Resistant Packaging

Walton W. W. 1982. An evaluation of the Poison Prevention Packaging Act. *Pediatrics* 69:363–70.

Clarke A., Walton W. W. 1979. Effect of safety packaging on aspirin ingestion by children. *Pediatrics*. 63:687–93.

Rodgers G. B. 2002. The effectiveness of child-resistant packaging for aspirin. *Arch Pediatr Adolesc Med*. 156:929–33.

Ginsburg M. J., O'Neill B., Baker S. P., Li G. 1991. *The Injury Fact Book*. 2nd ed. New York: Oxford University Press.

2.2. Hair Dryer Electrocutions

Budnick L. D. 1984. Bathtub-related electrocutions in the United States, 1979–1982. *JAMA*. 252:918–20.

CPSC saves lives through voluntary efforts and oversight: Making hair dryers safer. 1996. U.S. Consumer Product Safety Commission website. http://www.cpsc.gov/cpscpub/pubs/success/dryers.html. Updated 1996. Accessed February 2004.

Alan Schoem letter to importers and manufacturers of hair dryers. 2002. U.S. Consumer Product Safety Commission website. http://www.cpsc.gov/BUSINFO/Hairdryer.pdf. Updated November 25, 2002. Accessed February 2004.

2.3. Residential Smoke Detectors

National Firearm Protection Association. 2008. Fact sheets: Smoke alarms. http://www.nfpa.org/categoryList.asp?categoryID=278&URL=Research%20&%20Reports/Fact%20sheets/Fire%20protection%20equipment/Smoke%20alarms&cookie%5Ftest=1. Updated February 2008. Accessed March 2008.

Mallonee S. 2000. Evaluating injury prevention programs: The Oklahoma City smoke alarm project. *Future Child*. 10(1):164–74.

Haddix A. C., Mallonee S., Waxweiler R., Douglas, M. R. 2001. Cost effectiveness analysis of a smoke alarm giveaway program in Oklahoma City, Oklahoma. *Inj Prev*. 7:276–81.

Centers for Disease Control and Prevention. 1988. Perspectives in disease prevention and health promotion. *Morbidity and Mortality Weekly Report*, March 11, 37(9):138–49.

Home fire safety. 2008, Smoke alarms: What you need to know. U.S. Fire Administration website. http://www.usfa.fema.gov/public/hfs/alarms.shtm. Updated March 7, 2008. Accessed March 11, 2008.

Aherns, M. 1998. Batteries not included. *NFPA Journal*. May–June: 98–109.

McLoughlin E., Marchone M., Hanger L., German P. S., Baker S. P. 1985. Smoke detector legislation: Its effect on owner-occupied houses. *Am J Public Health*. 75:858–62.

2.4. Flammability of Children's Pajamas

McLoughlin E., Clarke N., Stahl K., Crawford J. D. 1977. One pediatric burn unit's experience with sleepwear-related injuries. *Pediatrics.* 60:405–9.

Knudson M. S., Bolieu S. L., Larson D. L. 1980. Children's sleepwear flammability standards: Have they worked? *Burns.* 6:255–60.

2.5. Tap Water Burns

Erdmann T. C., Feldman K. W., Rivara F. P., Heimbach D. M., Wall H. A. 1991. Tap water burn prevention: The effect of legislation. *Pediatrics.* 88:572–77.

Huyer D. W., Corkum S. H. 1997. Reducing the incidence of tap-water scalds: Strategies for physicians. *Can Med Assoc J.* 156:841–44.

Corkum S. 2000. Hot tap-water scalds. *Hospital for Sick Children Journal.* 2(4). http://www.sickkids.on.ca/journal/vol2issue4/hotwater.asp. Accessed March 2008.

2.6. Wringer Arm

MacCollum D. W. 1938. Wringer arm: A report of 26 cases. *N Engl J Med.* 218:549–54.

McCulloch J. H., Boswick J. A., Jonas R. 1973. Household wringer injuries: A three-year review. *J Trauma.* 13:1–8.

Warner B. L., Kenney B. D., Rice M. 2003. Washing machine related injuries: A continuing threat. *Inj Prev.* 9:357–60.

2.7. Infant Walkers

Thanks to Bob Dyer, who wrote an excellent student paper on this issue.

Shields B. J., Smith G. A. 2006. Success in the prevention of infant walker-related injuries: An nalysis of national data, 1990–2001. *Pediatrics.* 117(3): e452–e459.

Coats T. J., Allen M. 1991. Baby walker related injuries: A continuing problem. *Arch Emer Med.* 8:52–55.

Thein M. M., Lee J., Tay V., Ling S. L. 1997. Infant walker use, injuries, and motor development. *Inj Prev.* 3:63–66.

Kavanagh C. A., Banco L. 1982. The infant walker: A previously unrecognized health hazard. *Am J Dis Child.* 136:205–6.

Rodgers G. B., Leland E. W. 2005. An evaluation of the effectiveness of a baby walker safety standard to prevent stair-fall injuries. *J Safety Res.* 36:327–32.

2.8. Child Window Falls

Spiegel C. N., Lindaman F. C. 1977. Children Can't Fly: A program to prevent childhood morbidity and mortality from window falls. *Am J Public Health.* 67:1143–46.

Barlow B., Niemirska M., Gandhi R. P., Leblanc W. 1983. Ten years of experience with falls from a height in children. *J Pediatr Surg.* 18:509–11.

2.9. Child-Resistant Cigarette Lighters

Smith L. E., Greene M. A., Singh H. A. 2002. Study of the effectiveness of the U.S. safety standard for child resistant cigarette lighters. *Inj Prev.* 8:192–96.

CPSC and industry: Saving lives cost-effectively through cooperation. Child resistant cigarette lighters. 1996. U.S. Consumer Product Safety Commission website. http://www.cpsc.gov/cpscpub/pubs/success/lighters.html. Updated May 1996. Accessed February 2007.

New national standard for cigarette lighter. 1997. Australian Department of Consumer and Employer Protection website. http://www.docep.wa.gov.au/Corporate/Media/statements/1997/September/New_national_standar.html. Updated September 30, 1997. Accessed February 2007.

2.a. Jay Arena

Gifford J. 2004. Transcript, Jay Arena oral history interview, June 17. Duke Medical Center Archives website. http://archives.mc.duke.edu/programs/oh/oh_arena.html?view=body. Accessed March 2007.

Board of Health Promotion and Disease Prevention. 2004. *Forging a Poison Prevention and Control System.* Washington, DC: National Academies Press.

2.b. Bent Sorenson

Berger L. R., Mohan D. 1996. *Injury Control: A Global View.* New York: Oxford University Press.

Sorenson B. 1976. Prevention of burns and scalds in a developed country. *J Trauma.* 16:249–58.

2.c. Ken Feldman and Murray Katcher

Feldman K. W., Schaller R. T., Feldman J. A., McMillon M. 1977. Tap water scald burns in children. *Pediatrics.* 62:1–7.

Rivara F. P. 1998. Commentary: Tap water scald burns in children. *Pediatrics.* 102 (Suppl 1):256–58.

Katcher M. L. 1998. Tap water scale prevention: It's time for a worldwide effort. *Inj Prev.* 4:167–68.

National Committee for Injury Prevention and Control. 1989. *Injury Prevention: Meeting the Challenge.* New York: Oxford University Press.

2.d. Andrew McGuire

Trauma Foundation website. 2005. http://www.tf.org. Assessed June 2005.

Non-profit notables. 2004. Sonoma State University website. http://www.sonoma.edu/uaffairs/notables/nonprofit.html. Updated October 12, 2004. Assessed June 2005.

Fire-resistant cigarettes: Feasible but covered up. 1996. Center for Social Gerontology, Tobacco and the Elderly Project website. http://www.tcsg.org/tobacco/summer97/contentsss97.htm. Updated fall/winter 1996. Accessed June 2005.

3. WORK

Introduction

Centers for Disease Control and Prevention. 1999. Achievements in public health, 1900–1999: Improvements in workplace safety—United States. *Morbidity and Mortality Weekly Report,* June 11: 48:461–69.
1,001 safety success stories. 2007. U.S. Navy website. http://www.safetycenter. navy.mil/success/summaries.htm. Updated December 2007. Accessed March 2008.
The Zenith: Workers compensation specialists. 2005. Zenith Insurance Company website. http://www.thezenith.com/employers/Employers/page23399.html. Accessed June 2005.
Barss P. 1984. Injuries due to falling coconuts. *J Trauma.* 24:990–91.
Queensland invention stops falling coconuts. 2004. Australian Trade Commission website. http://www.austrade.gov.au/Queensland-invention-stops-falling-coconuts/default.aspx. Updated May 2004. Accessed June 2005.
Stout N. A., Jenkins E. L., Pizatella T. J. 1996. Occupational injury mortality rates in the United States: Changes from 1980 to 1989. *Am J Public Health.* 86:73–77.
Whiteside J. 1990. *Regulating Danger: The Struggle for Mine Safety in the Rocky Mountain Coal Industry.* Lincoln: University of Nebraska Press.
Stout N. A., Linn H. I. 2002. Occupational injury prevention research: Progress and priorities. *Inj Prev* 8:9–14.
Von Drehle D. 2003. *Triangle: The Fire That Changed America.* Boston: Atlantic Monthly Press.
Aldrich M. 1997. *Safety First: Technology, Labor and Business in the Building of American Work Safety: 1870–1939.* Baltimore: Johns Hopkins University Press.
Aldrich M. 2006. *Death Rode the Rails: American Railroad Accidents and Safety, 1828–1965.* Baltimore: Johns Hopkins University Press.
Geller E. S. 2001. *Working Safe: How to Help People Actively Care for Health and Safety.* 2nd ed. New York: Lewis Publishers.
U.S. Department of Labor, Bureau of Labor Statistics. 2008. Census of fatal occupational injuries. http://www.bls.gov/iif/oshcfoi1.htm. Updated February 2008. Accessed March 2008.
Leigh J. P., Markowitz S., Fahs M., Landrigan P. 2000. *Costs of Occupational Injuries and Illnesses.* Ann Arbor: University of Michigan Press.
Evans R. W., Evans R. I., Carvajal S., Perry S. 1996. A survey of injuries among Broadway performers. *Am J Public Health.* 86:77–80.
Cherniack M. G. 1992. Diseases of unusual occupations: An historical perspective. *Occup Med.* 7:369–84.

3.1. Phossy Jaw

Felton J. S. 1982. Classical syndromes in occupational medicine: Phosphorus necrosis—a classical occupational disease. *Am J Ind Med.* 3:77–120.
Raffle P. A. B., Lee W. R., McCallum R. I., Murray R. 1978. *Hunter's Diseases of Occupations.* 6th ed. London: Hodder & Stoughton.

Cherniack M. G. 1992. Diseases of unusual occupations: An historical perspective. *Occup Med.* 7:369–84.

Hamilton A. 1925. *The Industrial Poisons in the United States.* New York: Macmillan.

Myers M. L., McGlothlin J. D. 1996. Matchers' "phossy jaw" eradicated. *Am Ind Hyg Assoc J.* 57:330–33.

Hunter D. 1975. *The Diseases of Occupations.* 5th ed. Boston: Little, Brown.

3.2. Couplers, Brakes, and Trainmen

Aldrich M. 1997. *Safety First: Technology, Labor and Business in the Building of American Work Safety, 1870–1939.* Baltimore: Johns Hopkins University Press.

3.3. Building the Golden Gate Bridge

Adams C. F. 1987. *Heroes of the Golden Gate.* Palo Alto: Pacific Books.

Van Der Zee J. 1986. *The Gate: The True Story of the Design and Construction of the Golden Gate Bridge.* New York: Simon & Schuster.

Wonders of the world: Golden Gate Bridge. 2001. PBS website. http://www.pbs. org/wgbh/buildingbig/wonder/structure/golden_gate.html. Updated 2001. Accessed October 2005.

Golden Gate Bridge. 2005. Bridge Pros website. http://www.bridgepros.com/ projects/Goldengate/Golden_Gate.htm. Accessed October 2005.

Moran M. 2005. Suicide barrier sought for Golden Gate Bridge. *Psychiatr News.* 40(7):21. http://pn.psychiatryonline.org/cgi/content/full/40/7/21. Accessed October 2005.

3.4. Tractor Rollovers

Springfeldt B., Thorson J., Lee B. C. 1998. Sweden's thirty-year experience with tractor rollovers. *J Agric Saf Health.* 4:173–80.

Springfeldt B. 1998. Rollover. In International Labour Office, ed. *Encyclopedia of Occupational Health and Safety.* 4th ed. Hamilton, Canada: Canadian Centre for Occupational Health and Safety.

Reynolds S. J., Groves W. 2000. Effectiveness of roll-over protective structures in reducing farm tractor fatalities. *Am J Prev Med.* 18(suppl 4):63–69.

3.5. The Short-Handled Hoe

Thanks to Catherine Esquivel Pitti, who wrote an excellent student paper on this issue.

Murray D. L. 1982. The abolition of el cortito, the short-handled hoe: A case study in social conflict and state policy in California agriculture. *Soc Probl.* 30:26–39.

Ferris S., Sandoval R. 2006. The death of the short-handled hoe. http://www.pbs. org/itvs/fightfields/book1.html. Accessed June 2006.

Jourdane M. 2004. *The Struggle for Health and Legal Protection of Farm Workers: El Cortito.* Houston: Arte Publico Press.

3.6. Military Helicopter Fires

U.S. Department of Transportation, Federal Aviation Administration. 2002. *A Study of Helicopter Crash-Resistant Fuel Systems*. DOT/FAA/AR-01/76. Washington, DC: DOT, Federal Aviation Administration, February.

Hayden M. S., Shanahan D. F., Chen L. H., Baker S. P. 2005. Crash-resistant fuel system effectiveness in civil helicopter crashes. *Aviat Space Environ Med.* 76:782–85.

3.7. Needlestick Injuries

Dale J. C., Pruett S. K., Maker M. D. 1998. Accidental needlesticks in the phlebotomy service of the Department of Laboratory Medicine and Pathology at Mayo Clinic Rochester. *Mayo Clin Proc.* 73:611–15.

Zafar A. B., Butler C., Podgorny J. M., Mennonna P. A., Gaydos L. A., Sandiford J. A. 1997. Effect of a comprehensive program to reduce needlestick injuries. *Infect Control Hosp Epidemiol.* 18:712–15.

Rogers B., Goodno L. 2000. Evaluation of interventions to prevent needlestick injuries in health care occupations. *Am J Prev Med.* 18(suppl 4):90–98.

3.8. Firefighter Burns

Prezant D. J., Kelly K. J., Malley K. S., Karwa M. L., McLaughlin M. T., Hirschorn R., Brown A. 1999. Impact of a modern firefighting protective uniform on the incidence and severity of burn injuries in New York City firefighters. *J Occup Environ Med.* 41:469–79.

Ciampo M. N. 1998. Fabrics and fibers protecting the firefighter: Highly engineered nonwovens play an important role in defending NYC's "bravest." Nonwovens Industry website. http://www.nonwovens-industry.com/articles/1998/11/fabrics-and-fibers-protecting-the-firefighter. Updated November 1998. Accessed June 2004.

3.a. Samuel Plimsoll

Jones N. 2006. *The Plimsoll Sensation: The Great Campaign to Save Lives at Sea.* London: Little, Brown.

Samuel Plimsoll, M.P. 2007. Plimsoll Society website. http://www.plimsoll.com/history.html. Accessed February 2007.

Garfield S. 2006. The bottom line about Mr. Plimsoll (book review). *The Observer.* June 25.

Moorhouse J. 2006. The line of duty (book review). *The Guardian.* July 1.

The sailor's friend: Maritime history (book review). 2006. *The Economist.* July 6.

3.b. Alice Hamilton

Grant M. P. 1967. *Alice Hamilton: Pioneer Doctor in Industrial Medicine.* New York: Abelard-Schuman.

Alice Hamilton. 2005. National Women's Hall of Fame—Women of the Hall
    website. http://www.greatwomen.org/women.php?action=viewone&id=73.
    Accessed July 2005.
Hamilton A. 1985. *The Autobiography of Alice Hamilton, M.D., 1943*. Boston:
    Northeastern University Press.
Centers for Disease Control and Prevention. 1999. Alice Hamilton, M.D.
    Morbidity and Mortality Weekly Report, June 11, 48:462.
Rom W. V., ed. 1983. *Environmental and Occupational Medicine*. Boston:
    Little, Brown.

3.c. John Andrews

Felton J. S. 1982. Classical syndromes in occupational medicine: Phosphorus
    necrosis—a classical occupational disease. *Am J Ind Med.* 3:77–120.
Young A. N. 1982. Interpreting the dangerous trades: Workers' health in
    America and the career of Alice Hamilton, 1910–1935. PhD dissertation,
    Department of History, Brown University.
Progressive ideas. U.S. Department of Labor website. 2005. http://www.dol.
    gov/oasam/programs/history/mono-regsafepart06.htm. Accessed July 14, 2005.

3.d. Janine Jagger

Carlsen W. 1998. Virginia scientist leads fights to protect health care workers.
    SFGate.com (San Francisco Chronicle). April 14.
Feigenoff C. 2003. Macarthur Award for health care safety. University of
    Virginia Explorations website. http://oscar.virginia.edu/explorations/
    x8158.xml. Updated winter 2003. Accessed March 2007.
Jaggar J., Perry J. 2003. Comparisn of EPINet data for 1993 and 2001 shows
    marked decline in needlestick injury rates. *Advances in Exposure Prevention.*
    6:25–27.
Smith S. 2003. Leaders: Pointing the way to reducing needlestick injuries.
    Occupational Hazards website. http://www.occupationalhazards.com/
    Issue/Article/36503/Leaders_Pointing_the_Way_to_Reducing_Needlestick_
    Injuries.aspx. Updated July 28, 2003. Accessed March 2007.
Jagger J., Hunt E. H., Brand-Elnaggar J., Pearson R. D. 1998. Rates of needle-
    stick injury caused by various devices in a university hospital. *N Engl J Med.*
    319:284–88.
GSPH alum named Macarthur "genius." 2003. *University of Pittsburgh Alumni
    Magazine*. Spring: 24–25. http://www.publichealth.pitt.edu/docs/Public-
    Health-Sp03.pdf. Accessed March 2007.
Janine Jagger biographical sketch. 2007. University of Virginia Health System web-
    site. http://www.healthsystem.virginia.edu/internet/epinet/bio.cfm. Accessed
    March 2007.

3.e. Paul O'Neill

Arndt M. 2001. How O'Neill got Alcoa shining. *Business Week*. February 5.

Lagace M. 2002. Paul O'Neill: Values into action. Working Knowledge for Business Leaders. Harvard Business School website. http://hbswk.hbs.edu/archive/3159.html. Updated November 2, 2002. Accessed February 2008.

Smith S. 2002. America's safest companies. Occupational Hazards website. http://www.occupationalhazards.com/Issue/Article/35911/Americas_Safest_Companies_Part_One.aspx. Updated October 21, 2002. Accessed February 2008.

4. PLAY

Introduction

A comprehensive study of sports injuries in the U.S. 2003. American Sports Data website. http://www.americansportsdata.com/sports_injury1.asp. Updated June 2003. Accessed March 2008.

Hemenway D. 1993. *Prices and Choices: Microeconomic Vignettes.* 3rd ed. New York: University Press of America.

Solnick S. J., Calvert T. 1989. The grass is always greener: NFL injured reserve lists and type of field played on the previous week. Class paper, Harvard School of Public Health.

Janda D. H., Wojtys E. M., Hankin F. M. 1990. A three-phase analysis of the prevention of recreational softball injuries. *Am J Sports Med.* 18:632–35.

Hemenway D. 2006. *Private Guns, Public Health.* Ann Arbor: University of Michigan Press.

Holder H. D., Gruenewald P. J., Ponicki W. R., et al. 2000. Effect of community-based interventions on high-risk driving and alcohol-related injuries. *JAMA.* 284:2341–47.

4.1. Ski Boots and Bindings

Johnson R. J., Ettlinger C. F. 1982. Alpine ski injuries: Changes through the years. *Clin Sports Med.* 1:181–97.

Tapper E. M. 1978. Ski injuries from 1939 to 1976: The Sun Valley experience. *Am J Sports Med.* 6:114–21.

Gutman J., Weisbuch J., Wolf M. 1974. Ski injuries in 1972–1973. *JAMA.* 230:1423–25.

Sherry E., Fenelon L. 1991. Trends in skiing injury type and rates in Australia. *Med J Aust.* 155:513–15.

Ungerholm S., Engkvist O., Gierup J., Lindsjo U., Balkfors B. 1983. Skiing injuries in children and adults: A comparative study from an 8 year period. *Int J Sports Med.* 4:236–40.

4.2. Bicycle Helmets

Attewell R. G., Glase K., McFadden M. 2001. Bicycle helmet efficacy: A meta-analysis. *Accid Anal Prev.* 33:345–52.

Cameron M. H., Vulcan A. P., Finch C. F., Newstead S. V. 1994. Mandatory bicycle helmet use following a decade of helmet promotion in Victoria, Australia: An evaluation. *Accid Anal Prev.* 26:325–37.

Henderson M. 2005. The effectiveness of bicycle helmets: A review. Bicycle Helmet Safety Institute website. http://www.bhsi.org/henderso.htm. Updated June 2005. Accessed March 2008.

4.3. Hunter Orange

Cina S. J., Lariscy C. D., McGown S. T., et al. 1996. Firearm-related hunting fatalities in North Carolina: Impact of the "hunter orange" law. *South Med J.* 89:395–96.
Centers for Disease Control and Prevention. 1996. Hunting-associated injuries wearing "hunter orange" clothing: New York, 1989–1995. *Morbidity and Mortality Weekly Report,* 45:884–87.

4.4. Hockey Eye Injuries

Devenyi R. G., Pashby R. C., Pashby T. J. 1999. The hockey eye safety program. *Ophthalmol Clin North Am.* 12:359–66.
Dr. Tom Pashby Sports Safety Fund. 2004. http://www.drpashby.ca/content/fundaction.htm. Updated February 2004. Accessed March 2008.

4.5. Goalie Masks

Carter B. 2004. Plante changed goaltending. ESPN.com website. http://espn.go.com/classic/biography/s/Plante_Jacques.html. Updated February 2004. Accessed March 2008.
Carter B. 2004. More info on Jacques Plante. ESPN.com website. http://espn.go.com/classic/s/add_plante_jacques.html. Updated February 2004. Accessed March 2008.
History of masks. 2004. Painted Warriors website. http://users.aol.com/maskman30/historynf.html. Updated February 2004. Accessed March 2008.

4.6. Cervical Quadriplegia from Football Injuries

Torg J. S., Vegso J. J., Sennett B., et al. 1985. The national football head and neck injury registry: 14-year report on cervical quadriplegia, 1971 through 1984. *JAMA.* 254:3439–43.
Maroon J. C., Steele P. B., Berlin R. 1980. Football head and neck injuries: An update. *Clin Neurosurg.* 27:414–29.

4.7. Harvard Football

Park R. J. 2001. Mended or ended? Football injuries and the British and American medical press, 1870–1910. *Int J Hist Sport.* 18:110–33.
Nichols E. H., Richardson F. L. 1909. Football injuries of the Harvard squad for three years under the revised rules. *Boston Med Surg J.* 160:33–37.
Nichols E. H., Smith H. B. 1906. The physical aspect of American football. *Boston Med Surg J.* 154:1–8.

4.8. Broken Glass Lacerations

Baker M. D., Moore S. E., Wise P. H. 1986. The impact of the "bottle bill" legislation on the incidence of lacerations in childhood. *Am J Public Health.* 76:1243–44.

Baker M. D., Selbst S. M., Lanuti M. 1990. Lacerations in urban children. *Am J Dis Child.* 144:87–92.

Makary M. A. 1998. Reported incidence of injuries caused by street glass among urban children in Philadelphia. *Inj Prev.* 4:148–49.

4.9. Child Injuries in Harlem

Davidson L. L., Durkin M. S., Kuhn L., O'Connor P., Barlow B., Heagarty M. C. 1994. The impact of Safe Kids/Healthy Neighborhoods injury prevention program in Harlem, 1988 through 1991. *Am J Public Health.* 84:580–86.

Durkin M. S., Olesn S., Barlow B., Virella A., Connolly E. S. Jr. 1998. The epidemiology of urban pediatric neurological trauma: Evaluation of, and implications for, injury prevention programs. *Neurosurgery.* 42:300–310.

Durkin M. S., Laraque D., Lubman I., Barlow B. 1999. Epidemiology and prevention of traffic injuries to urban children and adolescents. *Pediatrics.* 103(6):e74. http://www.pediatrics.org/cgi/content/full/103/6/e74. Accessed March 18, 2008.

Howerton M. 1998. Safe kids in Harlem: Communities mobilize to prevent childhood injuries. *Children's Advocate.* March–April. http://4children.org/news/398harlm.htm. Accessed June 2005.

4.10. Playground Injuries

Howard A. W., MacArthur C., Willan A., Rothman L., Moses-McKeag A., MacPherson A. K. 2005. The effect of safer play equipment on playground injury rates among school children. *CMAJ.* 172:1443–46.

Norton C., Nixon J., Sibert J. R. 2004. Playground injuries to children. *Arch Dis Child.* 89:103–8.

4.11. Lawn Darts

Thanks to Catherine Hervouet-Zeiber and Molly Pretorius Holme, who wrote an excellent student paper on this issue.

Will G. F. 1988. Lawn darts and the limits of laissez-faire. *Washington Post.* May 8.

Sotiropoulos S. V., Jackson M. A., Tremblay G. F., Burry V. F., Olson L. C. 1990. Childhood lawn dart injuries: Summary of 75 patients and patient report. *Arch Pediatr Adolesc Med.* 144:980–82.

Bass J. 1988. Death, injuries prompt lawn dart ban. *United Press International.* October 28.

Bulletin! Government takes only 18 years to ban lawn darts! 1989. *Consumer Reports.* January 54(1):5.

4.12. Snowmobiling

Perrz J. J. 2003. Snowmobile injuries in North America. *Clin Orthop Relat Res.* 409:29–36.

National Trauma Registry report: Major injury in Canada, 2001–2002. 2004. Canadian Institute for Health Information website. http://secure.cihi.ca/cihiweb/dispPage.jsp?cw_page=media_15jan2003_2_e#report. Updated March 31, 2004. Accessed March 2008.

Rowe B. H., Therrien S. A., Bretzlaff J. A., Sahai V. S., Nagarajan K. V., Bota G. W. 1998. The effect of a community-based police surveillance program on snowmobile injuries and deaths. *Can J Public Health.* 89:57–61.

4.a. Tom Pashby

Hawthorn T. 2005. Tom Pashby, ophthalmologist. *Globe and Mail.* August 27.

Standards pioneer Dr. Tom Pashby passes away August 26, 2005. 2005. Canadian Standards Association Website. http://www.csa.ca/news/articles/default.asp?articleID=8519&language=english. Updated August 2005. Accessed March 2008.

4.b. Paul Vinger

McConnell G. 2004. Mission: Paintball safety. *Am Acad Pediatr News.* January, 24(1):17.

Foster C. S. 1996. Eye sports injuries. Ocular Immunology and Uveitis Foundation website. http://www.uveitis.org/patient/articles/articles/sports.html. Accessed March 2005.

Capao Filipe J. A. 2004. Soccer (football) ocular injuries: An important eye health problem. *Brit J Opthalmol.* 88:159–60.

Vinger P. 2000. A practical guide for sports eye protection. *Phys Sportsmed.* 28:1–13.

Hemenway D. 1974. *Industrywide Voluntary Product Standards.* Cambridge, MA: Ballinger.

4.c. Barbara Barlow

Howerton M. 1998. Safe kids in Harlem: Communities mobilize to prevent childhood injuries. *Children's Advocate.* March–April. http://4children.org/news/398harlm.htm. Accessed June 2005.

Q & A with Dr. Barbara Barlow. 2002. Allstate website. http://www.hsph.harvard.edu/research/hicrc/files/BarbaraBarlowInterview-Allstate.pdf. Updated 2002. Assessed June 2005.

A woman's crusade to help Harlem's children. 1995. *Columbia University Record.* 21(8). http://www.columbia.edu/cu/record/archives/vol21/vol21_iss8/record 2108.16.html.

Changing the face of medicine: Dr. Barbara Barlow. 2005. National Library of Medicine website. http://www.nlm.nih.gov/changingthefaceofmedicine/physicians/biography_22.html. Accessed June 2005.

Hellman P. 1995. Dr. Barbara Barlow, a guardian angel for the children. *Parade Magazine*. April 16.

Interview with Barbara Barlow. 2005. Robert Wood Johnson Foundation website. http://www.rwjf.org/files/newsroom/webcasts/InterviewBarbaraBarlow.pdf. Accessed June 2005.

5. NATURE

Introduction

Sheets B., Williams J. 2001. *Hurricane Watch: Forecasting the Deadliest Storms on Earth*. New York:Vintage Books.

National Weather Service website. 2005. http://www.weather.gov/om/hazstats. shtml. Accessed July 2005.

5.1. Icebergs

International Ice Patrol history. 2008. U.S. Coast Guard website. http://www.uscg.mil/hq/g%2Dep/history/HP_History.html. Updated March 2008. Accessed March 2008.

Pritchett, C. W. 1997. *Economic Value of the International Ice Patrol*. Groton, CT: U.S. Coast Guard Research and Development Center.

International Ice Patrol. 2008. U.S. Coast Guard website. http://www.uscg.mil/hq/g-cp/comrel/factfile/Factcards/InternationalIcePatrol.html. Accessed March 2008.

5.2. Hurricane Warnings

Sheets B., Williams J. 2001. *Hurricane Watch: Forecasting the Deadliest Storms on Earth*. New York:Vintage Books.

Jarrell J. D., Mayfield M., Rappaport E. N., Landsea C. W. 2001. The deadliest, costliest and most intense United States hurricanes from 1900 to 2000 (and other frequently requested hurricane facts). U.S. Dept. of Commerce, National Oceanic and Atmospheric Administration website. http://www.aoml.noaa.gov/hrd/Landsea/deadly/. Updated October 2001. Accessed March 2008.

The Weather Network. 2008. Tropical Storm Center. Hurricane preparedness. http://www.theweathernetwork.com/tropicalstorm/hurricane_preparedness. Accessed August 2008.

5.3. Volcano Evacuation

Newhall C.G. 2005. Benefits of volcano monitoring far outweigh costs: The case of Mount Pinatubo. U.S. Geological Survey website. http://pubs.usgs.gov/fs/1997/fs115-97/. Updated February 2005. Accessed March 2008.

Mount Pinatubo. 2005. Wikipedia Encyclopedia website. http://en.wikipedia.org/wiki/Pinatubo. Accessed August 2005.

Pinatubo volcano: The sleeping giant awakens. 1996. ABS-CBN Broadcasting Corporation website. http://park.org/Philippines/pinatubo/. Updated 1996. Accessed August 2005.

5.4. Tsunami Escape

Yalcinder A. C., Perincek D., Ersoy S., et al. 2005. December 26, 2004 Indian Ocean tsunami field survey at north of Sumatra island. UNESCO website. http://ioc.unesco.org/iosurveys/Indonesia/yalciner/yalciner.htm. Updated January 2005. Accessed January 2008.

Alifandi A. 2007. Saved by tsunami folklore. BBC News website. http://news.bbc.co.uk/1/hi/programmes/from_our_own_correspondent/6435979.stm. Broadcast March 10, 2007. Accessed January 2008.

5.5. Avalanche Transceivers

McIntosh S. E., Grissom C. K., Olivares C. R., Kim H. S., Tremper B. 2007. Cause of death in avalanche fatalities. *Wilderness Environ Med.* 18: 293–97.

Michahelles F., Ahonen T., Schiele B. 2003. Life increasing survival chances in avalanches by wearable sensors. In *Proceedings of the 3rd International Workshop on Smart Appliances and Wearable Computing, Providence, RI, May 19–22.* Washington, DC: International Workshop on Smart Appliances and Wearable Computing in collaboration with the IEEE Computer Society.

Hohlrieder M., Mair P., Wuertl, W., Brugger H. 2005. The impact of avalanche transceivers on morality from avalanche accidents. *High Alt Med Biol.* 6: 72–77.

McCammon I., Hageli P. 2007. Comparing avalanche decision frameworks using accident data from the United States. *Cold Regions Science and Technology.* 47:193–206.

Jamieson B. 1994. Transceivers and avalanche survival. *Avalanche News.* 42:8. http://www.schulich.ucalgary.ca/Civil/Avalanche/Papers/beacons_survival.pdf. Accessed February 2008.

Atkins D. 1998. Companion rescue and avalanche transceivers: The U.S. experience. Backcountry Access website. http://www.backcountryaccess.com/english/research/documents/CompanionRescue_Atkins.pdf. Updated 1998. Accessed February 2008.

Silverton N. A., McIntosh S. E., Kim H. S. 2007. Avalanche safety practices in Utah. *Wilderness Environ Med.* 18:264–70.

5.a. Benjamin Franklin

Adams C. F., ed. 1856. *The Works of John Adams, vol 1.* Boston: Little, Brown.

Herschbach D. Dr. Franklin's scientific amusements. *Harvard Magazine.* November 1995:36.

Isaacson W. 2003. *Benjamin Franklin: An American Life.* New York: Simon & Schuster.

Dray P. 2005. *Stealing God's Thunder: Benjamin Franklin's Lightning Rod and the Invention of America.* New York: Random House.

Cohen I. B. 1990. *Benjamin Franklin's Science.* Cambridge, MA: Harvard University Press.

5.b. William Redfield

Sheets B., Williams J. 2001. *Hurricane Watch: Forecasting the Deadliest Storms on Earth*. New York: Random House.
Nash J. M. 2006. Storm warnings. *Smithsonian Magazine*. September, 88–97.

6. VIOLENCE

Introduction

Vreeman R. C., Carroll A. E. 2007. A systematic review of school-based interventions to prevent bullying. *Arch Pediatr Adolesc Med*. 161:78–88.
Limbos M. A., Chan L. S., Warf C., Schneir A., Iverson E., Shekelle P., Kipke M. D. 2007. Effectiveness of interventions to prevent youth violence: A systematic review. *Am J Prev Med*. 33:65–74.
Zun L. S., Downey L. V., Rosen J. 2006. The effectiveness of an ED-based violence prevention program. *Am J Emerg Med*. 24:8–13.
Clarke R. V., Mayhew P. 1988. The British gas suicide story and its criminological implications. *Crime and Justice*. 10:79–116.
Clark R. V., Mayhew P. M. 1980. *Designing Out Crime*. London: HMSO.
Newman O. 1972. *Defensible Space: Crime Prevention through Urban Design*. New York: Macmillan.
Eck J. E. 2002. Preventing crime at places. In Sherman L. W., Farrington D. P., Welsh B. C., MacKenzie D. L., eds. *Evidence-Based Crime Prevention*. New York: Routledge.
Clarke R. V., ed. 1997. *Situations Crime Prevention: Successful Case Studies*. Guilderland, NY: Harrow & Heston.

6.1. Suicide in the Air Force

Knox K. L., Litts D. A., Talcott G. W., Feig J. C., Caine E. D. 2003. Risk of suicide and related adverse outcomes after exposure to a suicide prevention program in the U.S. Air Force: Cohort study. *Br Med J*. 327:1376–81.
U.S. Air Force. 2001. *The Air Force Suicide Prevention Program*. AFPAM 44–160. April.
Reducing suicide: A national imperative. 2002. Institute of Medicine, National Academy of Sciences website. http://www.nap.edu/books/0309083214/html/. Updated 2002. Accessed March 2008.

6.2. Suicide and Perestroika

Wasserman D., ed. 2001. *Suicide: An Unnecessary Death*. London: Martin Dunitz.
Wasserman D., Varnik A., Eklund G. 1994. Male suicides and alcohol consumption in the former USSR. *Acta Psychiatr Scand*. 89:306–13.
Wasserman D., Varnik A., Eklund G. 1998. Female suicides and alcohol consumption during perestroika in the former USSR. *Acta Psychiatr Scand*. 98 (suppl 394):26–33.

Wasserman D., Varnik A. 1998. Reliability of statistics on violent death and suicide in the former USSR, 1970–1990. *Acta Psychiatr Scand.* 98 (suppl 394): 34–41.

6.3. Gas Suicide in Britain

Clarke R. V., Mayhew P. 1989. Crime as opportunity: A note on domestic gas suicide in Britain and the Netherlands. *Br J Criminol.* 29:35–46.
Clarke R. V., Mayhew P. 1988. The British gas suicide story and its criminological implications. *Crime and Justice.* 10:79–116.
Hawton K., ed. 2005. Restriction of access to methods of suicide as a means of suicide prevention. In Hawton K., ed. *Prevention and Treatment of Suicidal Behavior.* New York: Oxford University Press.

6.4. Washington, DC, Metro

U.S. Department of Justice. 1997. *Visibility and Vigilance: Metro's Situational Approach to Preventing Subway Crime.* NCJ 166372. Washington, DC: Office of Justice Programs, National Institutes of Justice.
Clark R. V., ed. 1997. *Situational Crime Prevention: Successful Case Studies.* 2nd ed. New York: Harrow & Heston.

6.5. Nightclub Violence

Homel R., Hauritz M., Wortley R., McIlwain G., Carvolth R. 1997. Preventing alcohol-related crime through community action: The Surfers Paradise Safety Project. In Homel R., ed. *Policing for Prevention: Reducing Crime, Public Intoxication, and Injury.* New York: Criminal Justice Press, 35–90.
Hauritz M., Homel R., McIlwain G., Burrows T., Townsley M. 1998. Reducing violence in licensed venues: Community safety action projects. *Trends & Issues in Crime and Criminal Justice.* 101:1–6.
Homel R., Carvolth R., Hauritz M., McIlwain G., Teague R. 2004. Making licensed venues safer for patrons: What environmental factors should be the focus of interventions? *Drug Alcohol Rev.* 23:19–29.

6.6. Police Body Armor

U.S. Department of Justice. 2001. *Selection and Application Guide to Personal Body Armor.* NCJ 189633. Washington, DC: Office of Justice Programs, National Institutes of Justice.
Czarnecki F., Janowitz I. 2003. Ergonomics and safety in law enforcement. *Clin Occup Environ Med.* 3:399–417.

6.a. Thomas Mott Osborne

The Osborne family inventory text. 2008. New York Correction History website. http://www.correctionhistory.org/auburn&osborne/html/thomas-mottosbornebio-part1.html. Accessed February 2008.

Chamberlain R. W. 1935. *There Is No Truce: A Life of Thomas Mott Osborne*. New York: Macmillan.

Haasenritter D. K. 2003. The military correctional system: An overview. *Corrections Today*. December, 58–61.

Introduction by Frederick R.-L. Osbourne to Thomas Mott Osborne's *Within Prison Walls*. 1991. New York City Historical Society website. http://www. correctionhistory.org/auburn&osborne/tombrown/html/wpw_intro.html. Updated 1991. Accessed February 2008.

Thomas Mott Osborne. 2002. *UXL Encyclopedia of World Biography*. London: Gale Group.

6.b. Fathers Edward Flanagan and Gregory Boyle

Oursler F., Oursler W. 1949. *Father Flanagan of Boys Town*. Garden City, NY: Doubleday.

Fremon C. 1995. *Father Greg and the Homeboys: The Extraordinary Journal of Father Boyle and His Work with the Latino Gangs of East L.A.* New York: Hyperion.

Gross T. 2004. Father Gregory Boyle discusses his career working with former gang members in Los Angeles. Interview, *Fresh Air*, National Public Radio. February 17. http://www.religionandsocialpolicy.org/news/2-24-2004_ opinion_roundup.cfm. Accessed June 2005.

History. 2005. Girls and Boys Town website. http://www.girlsandboystown.org/. Accessed June 2005.

Boys Town USA. 2005. Center for Effective Collaboration and Practice website. http://cecp.air.org/resources/success/boystown.asp. Accessed June 2005.

Edward J. Flanagan. 2005. Wikipedia Encyclopedia website. http://en.wikipedia. org/wiki/Edward_J._Flanagan. Accessed June 2005.

Vasquez R. 2003. Hating gangs not the answer: Father Boyle calls for three-pronged approach to gangs. *La Prensa* (San Deigo). June 8. http://www. laprensa-sandiego.org/archieve/january17–03/gangs.htm. Accessed June 2005.

Homeboy Industries website. 2005. http://www.homeboy-industries.org. Accessed June 2005.

6.c. Erin Pizzey

Tjaden P., Thoennes N. 1998. *Prevalence, Incidence, and Consequences of Violence against Women*. NCJ 183781. Washington, DC: Office of Justice Programs, National Institute of Justice, U.S. Department of Justice.

Pizzey E. 1977. *Scream Quietly or the Neighbors Will Hear*. Short Hills, NJ: Ridley Enslow.

Herstory of domestic violence: A timeline of the battered women's movement. 1999. Minnesota Center against Violence and Abuse website. http://www. mincava.umn.edu/documents/herstory/herstory.html. Updated September 1999. Accessed January 2008.

7. MEDICAL TREATMENT

Introduction

Gabriel R. A., Metz K. S. 1992. *A History of Military Medicine. Vol. 1, From Ancient Times to the Middle Ages.* New York: Greenwood Press.

Pruitt B. A. Jr., Pruitt J. H., Davis J. H. History. In Moore E. E., Feliciano D. V., Mattox K. L., eds. 2003. *Trauma.* 5th ed. New York: McGraw Hill.

Greenwood J. T., Berry F. C. 2005. *Medics at War: Military Medicine from Colonial Times to the 21st Century.* Annapolis, MD: Naval Institute Press.

Rutkow I. M. 2005. *Bleeding in Blue and Gray: Civil War Surgery and the Evolution of American Medicine.* New York: Random House.

Oliver C. 2001. Trauma: History. In Lock S., Last J., Dunea G., eds. *The Oxford Illustrated Companion to Medicine.* New York: Oxford University Press.

Rich N. M., Burris D. G. 2005. Modern military surgery: 19th century compared with 20th century. *J Am Coll Surg.* 200:321–22.

Pruitt B. A. 2006. Combat casualty care and surgical progress. *Ann Surg.* 243:715–29.

Foss J. 1989. A history of trauma care: From cutter to trauma surgeon. *AORN J.* 50:21–30.

Gawande A. 2007a. *Better: A Surgeon's Notes on Performance.* New York: Henry Holt.

Liberman M., Mulder D. S., Sampalis J. S. 2004. The history of trauma care systems from Homer to telemedicine. *McGill J Med.* 7:214–22. http://www.medicine.mcgill.ca/mjm/issues/v07n02/feature_rev/feature_rev.htm. Accessed April 2008.

Gawande A. 2007b. The checklist. *New Yorker.* December 10, 86–101.

Pronovost P., Needham D., Berenholtz S., et al. 2006. An intervention to decrease catheter-related bloodstream infections in the ICU. *N Engl J Med.* 355:2725–32.

Trunkey D. D. 2000. History and development of trauma care in the United States. *Clin Orthop Relat Res.* 374:36–46.

Trunkey D. D., Ochsner M. G. Jr. 1995. Management of battle casualties. In Feliciano D. V., Moore E. E., Mattox K. L., eds. *Trauma.* 3rd ed. Stamford, CT: Appleton & Lange, 1023–35.

David J. H. History of trauma. 1995. In Feliciano D. V., Moore E. E., Mattox K. L., eds. *Trauma.* 3rd ed. Stamford, CT: Appleton & Lange, 3–13.

7.1. Acute Care for Burn Injury

Wolf S. E., Rose J. K., Desai M. H., Mileski J. P., Barrow R. E., Herndon D. 1997. Mortality determinants in massive pediatric burns. *Ann Surg.* 225:554–69.

Saffle J. R. 1998. Predicting outcomes of burns. *N Engl J Med.* 338:387–88.

Sheridan R. L., Hinson M. I., Liang M. H., Nackel A. F., Schoenfeld D. A., Ryan C. M., Mulligan J. L. 2000. Long term outcome of children surviving massive burns. *JAMA.* 283:69–73.

O'Neill J. A. Jr. 2000. Advances in the management of pediatric trauma. *Am J Surg.* 180:365–69.

7.2. Trauma Systems

Mann N. C., Mullins R. J., MacKenzie E. J., Jurkovich G. J., Mock C. N. 1999. Systematic review of published evidence regarding trauma system effectiveness. *J Trauma.* 47(suppl 3):S:25–33.

Miller T. R., Levy D. T. 1995. The effect of regional trauma care systems on costs. *Arch Surg.* 130:188–93.

Shackford S. R., Hollingworth-Fridlund P., Cooper G. F., Eastman A. B. 1986. The effect of regionalization upon the quality of trauma care as assessed by concurrent audit before and after institution of a trauma system: A preliminary report. *J Trauma.* 26:812–20.

7.3. Anesthesia

Institute of Medicine. 2000. *To Err Is Human: Building a Safer Health System.* Washington, DC: National Academy Press.

Ziegler J. 2000. A medical specialty blazes a trail. *Accelerating Change Today for America's Health.* February:26–28.

Cooper J. B. 2001. Accidents and mishaps in anesthesia: How they occur; how to prevent them. *Minerva Anestesiol.* 67:310–13.

7.4. The Jaipur Foot

McGirk T. 2008. Heroes of medicine: The global scourge of land mines left thousands limbless and then two gifted Indians developed the $28 foot. *Time* Website. http://www.time.com/time/reports/heroes/foot.html. Accessed February 2008.

Dr. Pramod Karan Sethi obituary: Surgeon who devised a cheap prosthetic limb that helps poor amputees around the world. 2008. Times Online website. http://www.timesonline.co.uk/tol/comment/obituaries/article3185855.ece. Updated January 15, 2008. Accessed February 2008.

Serlin D. 2001. The clean room: Making the Jaipur foot. *Cabinet Magazine Online.* Fall. http://www.cabinetmagazine.org/issues/4/jaipurfoot.php. Accessed February 2008.

Srinivasan R. 2002. Technology sits cross-legged: Developing the Jaipur foot prosthesis. In Ott K., Serlin D., Mihm S., eds. *Artificial Parts, Practical Lives: Modern Histories of Prosthetics.* New York: New York University Press, 327–47.

7.a. Baron Larrey

Thanks to Christine Sison and Jacob Joy, who wrote an excellent student paper on this hero.

Faria M. A. 1990. Dominique-Jean Larrey: Napoleon's surgeon from Egypt to Waterloo. *J Med Assoc Ga.* 79:693–95.

Skandalakis P. N., Panagiotis L., Zoras O., Skandalakis J. E., Mirilas P. 2006. "To afford the wounded speedy assistance": Dominique Jean Larrey and Napoleon. *World J Surg.* 30:1392–99.

Dr. Dominique-Jean Larrey, surgeon-in-chief of Napoleon's army. 2006. Napoleonic Society website. http://www.napoleonicsociety.com/english/ LarreyJean.htm. Accessed June 2006.

Crumplin M. K. 2002. Surgery in the Napoleonic wars. *J R Coll Surg Edinb.* 47:566–78.

Feinsod M. 1998. The surgeon and the emperor: A humanitarian on the battle-field. *Harefuah.* 135:340–43.

Ortiz J. M. 1998. The revolutionary flying ambulance of Napoleon's surgeon. *U.S. Army Medical Department Journal.* October, 17–25.

Brewer L. A. 1986. Baron Dominique Jean Larrey (1176–1842): Father of modern military surgery, innovator, humanist. *J Thorac Cardiovasc Surg.* 92:1096–98.

Bodemer C. W. 1982. Baron Dominique Jean Larrey, Napoleon's surgeon. *Bull Am Coll Surg.* July 18–21.

Richardson R. G. 1974. *Larrey: Surgeon to Napoleon's Imperial Guard.* London: John Murray.

7.b. Florence Nightingale

Dossey B. M. 1999. *Florence Nightingale: Mystic, Visionary, Healer.* Springhouse, PA: Springhouse.

Florence Nightingale. 2008. Wikipedia Encyclopedia website. http://en.wikipedia. org/wiki/Florence_Nightingale. Accessed February 2008.

Gill C. J., Gill G. C. 2005. Nightingale in Scutari: Her legacy reexamined. *Clin Infect Dis.* 40:1799–805.

Small H. 1999. *Florence Nightingale: Avenging Angel.* New York: Palgrave Macmillan.

Strachey L. 2006. *Eminent Victorians.* Mineola, NY: Dover.

Audain C. 2005. Florence Nightingale. Agnes Scott College website. http://www.agnesscott.edu/lriddle/women/nitegale.htm. Accessed June 2005.

7.c. Peter Safar

Mitka M. 2003. Peter J. Safar, MD: Father of CPR, innovator, teacher, humanist. *JAMA.* 289:2485–86.

Pretto E. A. Jr. 2005. Witness to a wonderful life. *Prehosp Disaster Med.* 20:82–84.

Srikameswaran A. 2002. Dr. Peter Safar: A life devoted to cheating death. *Pittsburgh Post-Gazette.* March 31. http://www.post-gazette.com/lifestyle/ 20020331safar0331fnp2.asp. Accessed March 2007.

Srikameswaran A. 2003. Obituary: Dr. Peter Safar, renowned Pitt physician called father of CPR. *Pittsburgh Post-Gazette.* August 5. http://www.post-gazette. com/obituaries/20030805safar0805p1.asp. Accessed March 2007.

Safar P. 1958. Ventilatory efficacy of mouth-to-mouth artificial respiration. *JAMA.* 167:335–41.

7.d. Jeffrey Cooper and Ellison (Jeep) Pierce

Cooper receives AANA Award. 2003. Anesthesia Patient Safety Foundation, APSF Newsletter website. http://www.apsf.org/resource_center/newsletter/2003/fall/03cooper.htm. Updated Fall 2003. Accessed August 2005.

Cooper J. B., Newbower R. S., Long C. D., McPeek M. 1978. Preventable anesthesia mishaps: A study of human factors. *Anesthesiology.* 49:399–406.

Gawande A. 2002. *Complications: A Surgeon's Note on an Imperfect Science.* New York: Henry Holt.

Parsons D. W. 2000. Federal legislation efforts to improve patient safety. *Eff Clin Pract.* November/December. http://www.acponline.org/journals/ecp/novdec00/parsons.htm. Accessed March 2008.

7.e. Lucian Leape

Leape L. L., Askcraft K. W., Scarpelli D. G., Holder T. M. 1971. Hazard to health: Liquid lye. *N Engl J Med.* 284:578–81.

Herman R. 2000. The human factor. *Harvard Public Health Review.* Fall, 24–31.

Wachter R. 2007. In conversation with Lucian Leape, MD. AHRQ Morbidity and Mortality Rounds on the Web. http://www.webmm.ahrq.gov/perspective.aspx?perspectiveID=28. Accessed August 2007.

Leape L. L. 1994. Error in medicine. *JAMA.* 272:1851–57.

7.f. Subroto Das

Leading social entrepreneurs: Subroto Das. 2006. Ashoka website. http://ashoka.org/node/2637. Updated 2006. Accessed March 2007.

Indian doctor's road safety revolution. 2004. BBC News website. http://news.bbc.co.uk/2/hi/south_asia/3934177.stm. Updated August 8, 2004. Accessed May 2007.

Rao R. 2004. Tracking road accidents. Tribune Online website. http://www.tribuneindia.com/2004/20040806/science.htm#1. Updated August 6, 2004. Accessed May 2007.

8. MODELS

8.1. Industry: Airlines

Mitchell M. L., Maloney M. T. 1989. Crisis in the cockpit? The role of market forces in promoting air travel safety. *J Law Econ.* 32:329–55.

Hemenway D. 1993. Injury prevention. In Hemenway D. *Prices and Choices.* Lanham, MD: University Press of America.

Institute of Medicine. 2000. *To Err Is Human: Building a Safer Health System.* Washington, DC: National Academy Press.

Lacey R. O. 2007. Organizational politics of prevention. University of California, Irvine, Center for Organizational Research website. http://www.cor.web.uci.edu/ufiles/calendar/Lacey_COR_PoliticsPrevention.pdf. Accessed April 2007.

Tamuz M. 2007. Understanding accident precursors. In *Accident Precursor Analysis and Management*. Washington, DC: National Academy of Engineering, National Academies Press. http://www.nae.edu/NAE/engecocom.nsf/0754c87f163f599e85256ccaoo588f49/85256cfb004759c185256dd60053b88d/$FILE/Tamuz.PDF. Accessed April 2007.

Helmreich R. L. 2000. On error management: Lessons from aviation. *Br Med J*. 320:781–85.

Borowsky M., Gaynor J. 2007. What's more dangerous? Airplane versus automobile accidents. Statistics and Mathematics Department, U.S. Naval Safety Center. http://findarticles.com/p/articles/mi_moFKE/is_4_47/ai_86504189. Accessed August 2007.

Safety record of U.S. air carriers. 2007. Air Transport Association website. http://www.airlines.org/economics/specialtopics/SafetyRecordOfCarriers.htm. Accessed April 2007.

8.2. Town: Harstad, Norway

Ytterstad B. 1995. The Harstad injury prevention study: Hospital-based injury recording used for outcome evaluation of community-based prevention of bicyclist and pedestrian injury. *Scand J Prim Health Care*. 13:141–49.

Ytterstad B., Wasmuth H. H. 1995. The Harstad injury prevention study: Evaluation of hospital-based injury recording and community-based intervention for traffic injury prevention. *Accid Anal Prev*. 27:111–23.

Ytterstad B., Sogaard A. J. 1995. The Harstad injury prevention study: Prevention of burns in small children by a community-based intervention. *Burns*. 21:259–66.

Ytterstad B. 1996. The Harstad injury prevention study: Community based prevention of fall-fractures in the elderly evaluated by means of a hospital-based injury recording system in Norway. *J Epidemiol Community Health*. 50:551–58.

Ytterstad B. 1996. The Harstad injury prevention study: The epidemiology of sports injuries. *Br J Sports Med*. 30:64–68.

Ytterstad B., Smith G. S., Coggar C. A. 1998. Harstad injury prevention study: Prevention of burns in young children by community-based intervention. *Inj Prev*. 4:176–80.

Ytterstad B. 2003. The Harstad injury prevention study: A decade of community-based traffic injury prevention with emphasis on children. *Int J Circumpolar Health*. 62:61–74.

8.3. City: Boston and Youth Homicide

Pruitt B. H. 2001. The Boston strategy: A story of unlikely alliances. Boston Strategy website. http://sasnet.com/bostonstrategy/story.html. Updated 2001. Accessed March 2008.

Kennedy D. M., Piehl A. M., Braga A. A. 1996. Youth violence in Boston: Gun markets, serious youth offenders, and a use-reduction strategy. *Law Contemp Prob*. 59:147–96.

Hemenway D., Prothrow-Stith D., Bergstein J. M., Ander R., Kennedy B. P. 1996. Gun carrying among adolescents. *Law Contemp Prob.* 59:39–53.

Braga A. A., Kennedy D. M., Waring E. J., Piehl A. M. 2001. Problem-oriented policing, deterrence, and youth violence: An evaluation of Boston's Operation Ceasefire. *J Res Crime Delinq.* 38:195–225.

Piehl A. M., Kennedy D. M., Braga A. A. 2000. Problem solving and youth violence: An evaluation of the Boston Gun Project. *Am Law Econ Rev.* 60: 58–106.

Hampson R. 2007. Gang peacemaker's death imperils truce in Boston. *USA Today* website. http://www.usatoday.com/printedition/news/20070306/1a_cover06.art.htm. Updated March 5, 2007. Accessed August 2007.

Slack D. 2007. Antigang workers face uphill climb: Street unit's mission, makeup shifted. *Boston Globe* website. http://www.boston.com/news/local/articles/2007/07/19/antigang_workers_face_uphill_climb/. Updated July 19, 2007. Accessed August 2007.

8.4. Country: Sweden

A league table of child deaths by injury in rich countries, 2001. 2001.UNICEF website. http://www.unicef-icdc.org/publications/pdf/repcard2e.pdf. Accessed August 2007.

Jansson B., Ponce de Leon A., Ahmed N., Jansson V. 2006. Why does Sweden have the lowest childhood injury mortality in the world? The role of architecture and public pre-school services. *J Public Health Policy.* 27: 146–65.

Sweden: Progress on Regional Priority Goal II on accidents, injuries and physical activity. 2006. European Environment and Health Committee website. http://www.euro.who.int/eehc/implementation/20060713_1. Accessed August 2007.

Ekman R., Svanstrom L., Langberg B. 2005. Temporal trends, gender, and geographic distributions in child and youth injury rates in Sweden. *Inj Prev.* 11:29–32.

Bergstein A. B., Rivara F. P. 1991. Sweden's experience in reducing childhood injuries. *Pediatrics.* 88:69–74.

Berfenstam R. 1995. Sweden's pioneering child accident programme: 40 years later. *Inj Prev.* 1:68–69.

Berfenstam R. 1977. Learning from Sweden's experiences in preventing childhood accidents. *Pediatr Ann.* 6:742–51.

8.5. Country: The Netherlands

Pucher J., Dijkstra L. 2003. Promoting safe walking and cycling to improve public health: Lessons from the Netherlands and Germany. *Am J Public Health.* 93:1509–16.

Nicole M. 2006. A short history of pedestrian safety policies in Western Europe. ICTCT website. http://www.ictct.org/workshops/07-Beijing/3_4Muhlrad 138_149.pdf. Updated 2006. Accessed August 2007.

9. FUTURE SUCCESSES

9.1. Speed

Evans L. 2004. *Traffic Safety*. Bloomfield Hills, MI: Science Serving Society.

National Highway Traffic Safety Administration. 1984. *A Decade of Experience Evaluates the Benefits and Costs of the 55 mph Speed Limit and Assesses the Effectiveness of State Laws in Inducing Compliance*. HS-038 162.Washington, DC: Transportation Research Board.

Research and statistics Q&A, speed and speed limits. 2007. Insurance Institute of Highway Safety website. http://www.iihs.org/research/qanda/speed_limits.html. Accessed May 2007.

Greenstone M. 2002. A reexamination of resource allocation responses to the 65 mph speed limit. *Economic Inquiry*. 40:271–78.

Garber S., Graham J. D. 1990. The effect of the new 65 mph speed limit on rural highway fatalities: A state-by-state analysis. *Accid Anal Prev*. 22:137–49.

Centers for Disease Control and Prevention. 1994. Risky driving behaviors among teenagers: Gwinnett County, Georgia. 1993. *Morbidity and Mortality Weekly Report*. June 10, 43(22):405–9.

Lewis L. 2005. *It's No Accident: The Real Story behind the Senseless Death and Injury on Our Roads*. Washington, DC: Partnership for Safe Driving.

Compton R. P. 2005. Speeding: Who, when, where. DOT HS 809 963. Paper presented at the National Forum on Speeding, Washington, DC, June 15–16.

Police pursuit in pursuit of policy. 1992. Illinois State University Department of Criminal Justice website. http://www.geocities.com/bears_in_the_air/policepursuit.html. Updated 1992. Accessed March 2008.

Hill J. 2002. High-speed police pursuits: Dangers, dynamics and risk reduction. *FBI Law Enforcement Bulletin*. July, 71 (7):14–18.

McCartt A. T. 2007. Letter to the National Highway Traffic Safety Administration and the Federal Motor Carrier Safety Administration. Insurance Institute for Highway Safety website. http://www.iihs.org/laws/comments/pdf/nhtsa_fmcsa_ds_atm_032707.pdf. Updated March 27, 2007. Accessed May 2007.

Teed N., Lund A. K., Knoblauch R. 1993. The duration of speed reductions attributable to radar detectors. *Accid Anal Prev*. 25:131–37.

Raymond M. 2002. Penumbral crimes. *Am Crim Law Rev*. Fall, 39(45):1395.

9.2. Sports

Janda D. H. 2003a. *The Awakening of a Surgeon*. Ann Arbor, MI: Institute for Preventative Sports Medicine.

Janda D. H. 2003b. The prevention of baseball and softball injuries. *Clin Orthop Relat Res*. 409:20–28.

Janda D. H., Wojtys E. M., Hankin F. M., Benedict M. E. 1988. Softball sliding injuries: A prospective study comparing standard and modified bases. *JAMA*. 259:1848–50.

Janda D. H., Wojtys E. M., Hankin F. M., et al. 1990. A three-phase analysis of the prevention of recreational softball injuries. *Am J Sports Med*. 18:632–35.

Janda D. H., Maguire R., Mackesy D., et al. 1993. Sliding injuries in college and professional baseball. *Clin J Sport Med.* 3:78–81.

Dick R., Sauers E. L., Agel J., et al. 2007. Descriptive epidemiology of collegiate men's baseball injuries: National Collegiate Athletic Association Injury Surveillance System, 1988–1989 through 2003–2004. *J Athl Train.* 42:183–93.

Greenwald R. M., Penna L. H., Crisco J. J. 2001. Differences in batted ball speed with wood and aluminum baseball bats: A batting cage study. *J Appl Biomech.* August, 17(3):241–52.

Keteyian A. 2002. Bats should crack, not skulls. *Sporting News* website. http://findarticles.com/p/articles/mi_m1208/is_25_226/ai_95765251. Updated June 24, 2002. Accessed May 2007.

Adelson E. 2000. Bat controversy lingers over NCAA. ESPN.com website. http://www.espn.go.com/gen/s/2000/0329/453294.html. Updated March 29, 2000. Accessed May 2007.

Ritter J. 2007. Aluminum bat backlash. *Beacon News* (Aurora, IL). May 13.

McDowell M., Ciocco M. V. 2006. A pitcher injury risk assessment study analyzing composite, titanium, aluminum and wood softball bat performance. *Eur J Sports Sci.* 6:155–62.

Caine D. J., Caine C. G., Lindner K. J., eds. 1996. *Epidemiology of Sports Injuries.* Champaign, IL: Human Kenetics.

Hootman J. M., Dick R., Angel J. 2007. Epidemiology of collegiate injuries for 15 sports: Summary and recommendations for injury prevention. *J Athl Train.* 42:311–19.

Ekstrand J., Gillquist J., Liljedahl S. 1983. Prevention of soccer injuries. *Am J Sports Med.* 11:116–20.

9.3. Suicide

Friend T. 2003. Jumpers: The fatal grandeur of the Golden Gate Bridge. *New Yorker.* October 13, 48–59.

Miller M., Azrael D., Hemenway D. 2006. Belief in the inevitability of suicide: Results from a national survey. *Suicide Life Threat Behav.* 36:1–11.

Owens D., Horrocks J., House A. 2002. Fatal and non-fatal repetition of self-harm. *Br J Psychiatry.* 181:193–99.

Seiden R. H. 1978. Where are they now? A follow-up study of suicide attempters from the Golden Gate Bridge. *Suicide Life Threat Behav.* 8:203–16.

Lester D. 1993. Suicide from bridges in Washington, D.C. *Percept Mot Skills.* 77:534.

Bennewith O., Nowers M., Gunnell D. 2007. Effect of barriers on the Clifton suspension bridge, England, on local patterns of suicide: Implications for prevention. *Br J Psychiatry.* 190:266–67.

Pelletier A. R. 2007. Preventing suicide by jumping: The effect of a bridge safety fence. *Inj Prev.* 13:57–59.

Beautrais A. L. 2001. Effectiveness of barriers at suicide jumping sites: A case study. *Aust N Z J Psychiatry.* 35:557–62.

Guthmann E. 2005. The allure: Beauty and an easy route to death have long made the Golden Gate Bridge a magnet for suicides. *San Francisco Chronicle.* October 30.

Hendin H. 1995. *Suicide in America.* New York: Norton.

9.4. Shootings

Centers for Disease Control and Prevention. 1997. Rates of homicide, suicide and firearm-related death among children: Twenty-six industrialized countries. *Morbidity and Mortality Weekly Report,* February 7:101–5.

Hemenway D. 2006. *Private Guns, Public Health.* Ann Arbor: University of Michigan Press.

Miller M., Azrael D., Hemenway D. 2007a. State-level homicide victimization rates in the U.S. in relation to survey measures of household firearm ownership, 2001–2003. *Soc Sci Med.* 64:656–64.

Miller M., Lippmann S. J., Azrael D., Hemenway D. 2007b. Household firearm ownership and rates of suicide across the 50 states. *J Trauma.* 62:1029–35.

Minimum age to purchase and possess firearms. 2006. Legal Community Against Violence website. http://www.lcav.org/content/minimum_age_purchase_possess.pdf. Updated August 2006. Accessed August 2007.

Hemenway D., Prothrow-Stith D., Bergstein J. M., Ander R., Kennedy B. P. 1996. Gun carrying among adolescents. *Law Contemp Prob.* 59:39–53.

Hemenway D., Miller M. 2004. Gun threats against and self-defense gun use by California adolescents. *Arch Pediatr Adolesc Med.* 158:395–400.

Hemenway D. 2006. The public health approach to reducing firearm injury and violence. *Stanford Law Policy Rev.* 17:635–56.

10. SUMMARY

Introduction

Institute of Medicine. 1988. *The Future of Public Health.* Washington, DC: National Academy Press.

Isaacs S. L., Schroeder S. A. 2001. Where the public good prevails: Lessons from success stories in health. *American Prospect.* June 4, 26–30.

Waller J. A. 1994. Reflections on a half-century of injury control. *Am J Public Health.* 84:664–70.

Baker S. 1997. Advances and adventures in trauma prevention. *J Trauma.* 42:369–73.

Garrett L. 2000. *Betrayal of Trust: The Collapse of Global Public Health.* New York: Hyperion.

Hale A. R., Glendon A. I. 1987. *Individual Behavior in the Control of Danger.* New York: Elsevier.

Success Stories

Gielen A. C., Sleet D. A., DiClemente R. J. 2006. *Injury and Violence Prevention: Behavioral Science Theories, Methods, and Applications.* San Francisco: Jossey-Bass.

National Research Council. 2005. *Firearms and Violence: A Critical Review.* Washington, DC: National Academy Press.

Hale A. R., Glendon A. I. 1987. *Individual Behavior in the Control of Danger.* New York: Elsevier.

Conclusion

Salinger J. D. 1951. *Catcher in the Rye.* Boston: Little, Brown.

APPENDIX: SCIENTIFIC INJURY STUDIES

National Research Council. 1985. *Injury in America: A Continuing Public Health Problem.* Washington, DC: National Academy Press.

Institute of Medicine. 1999. *Reducing the Burden of Injury: Advancing Prevention and Treatment.* Washington, DC: National Academy Press.

Pless I. B. 2006. A brief history of injury and accident prevention publications. *Inj Prev.* 12:65–66.

Rosenberg M. L., Hammond R. 1998. Surveillance the key to firearm injury prevention. *Am J Prev Med.* 15(suppl 3):1.

Foege B. J. 1996. Foreword. In Murray C. J. L., Lopez A. D., eds. *The Global Burden of Disease.* Cambridge, MA: Harvard University Press, xxv–xxvi.

Index

Text: 10/13 Sabon
Display: Sabon
Compositor: International Typesetting and Composition
Printer and Binder: Maple-Vail Book Manufacturing Group